D0938454

That's How

the Light

Gets In

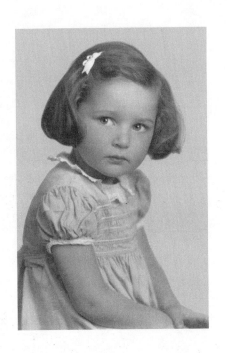

That's How the Light Gets In

MEMOIR of a PSYCHIATRIST

Susan Rako, M.D.

 HARMONY BOOKS / *New York*

Published in the United States by Harmony Books, an imprint of the Crown
Publishing Group, a division of Random House, Inc., New York.
www.crownpublishing.com

Harmony Books is a registered trademark and the Harmony Books colophon is
a trademark of Random House, Inc.

Library of Congress Cataloging-in-Publication Data
Rako, Susan.
That's how the light gets in : memoir of a psychiatrist / Susan Rako.—1st ed.
Includes bibliographical references.
1. Rako, Susan.   2. Women psychiatrists—United States—Biography.
    [DNLM: 1. Rako, Susan.   2. Psychiatry—United States—
    Personal Narratives.]   I. Title.
RC438.6R35A3 2005
616.89'0092—dc22   2004029885

ISBN 1-4000-4605-X

Printed in the United States of America

Design by Ruth Lee-Mui

10 9 8 7 6 5 4 3 2 1

First Edition

To my granddaughter,

ALEXANDRA GRACE,

*whose delight in life, innocence,
and brilliant intelligence
inspire joy, love, compassion, and awe*

*And to her extraordinary mother,
my beloved daughter,*

JENNIFER

ACKNOWLEDGMENTS

I am grateful to my parents, who nourished me in all the ways they could, and who, beyond these limits, supplied grit in the oyster, having endowed me with the stuff of which pearl is made.

My heartfelt appreciation to Jennifer S. Rako, Jeanne Mayell, Deborah Rose, Elissa Arons, Linda Herman Land, Marie Mantos Harburger, Ruth Hapgood, and to others who know my gratitude for their dependable support and wisdom.

I bless the day I met my editor and friend, Shaye Areheart, whom I thank for her commitment to this book and for setting me up with another editing genius, Kim Kanner Meisner—whose respectful and brilliant editorial suggestions gave me the will to go deeper.

AUTHOR'S NOTE

The events described in this memoir are true.
The persons portrayed are real.
The names of some of the individuals
have been changed to protect their privacy
or the privacy of their families.

CONTENTS

Contents

There is a crack, a crack in everything.
That's how the light gets in.

LEONARD COHEN
"Anthem"

*That's How
the Light
Gets In*

Preface

When Freud said, of the goal of psychoanalysis, "Where id was, there ego shall be," he meant that through knowledge of oneself, one's urges, one's longings, a person lessens the risk of being unconsciously driven by them. Clearly, being on to oneself is the foundation for responsible existence. But *existence* is the operational word here. I say: Where ego is, there tedium shall be. It takes getting beyond oneself, free of self-consciousness, to be *alive*. Creative experience happens in this space. Remarkably, when we are caught up in living beyond the *me* filter, we often lose track of the passage of time.

In my childhood, I lived in this sense mainly while reading books. Dependably carried beyond any troublesome focus on myself, whenever I could, I read until I was dizzy and my cheeks were hot and red. Coming out of the world of the book at the end of a Saturday afternoon was like stepping down from living to existing. There were a few other, too infrequent experiences that took me out of myself during my childhood. These were, for the most part, times spent in nature and away from home tensions—feeding the carp at Green Hill Park alone with my father, walking the sands and jetties of Cape Cod when I vacationed for a summer week with my aunt and uncle.

Curiously, when I was twenty-two (in 1961) I felt the

urge to write "a book of wisdom" (the stiff phrase that unaccountably came to mind at the time). I tried to write, scraped around, and came up with two possible topics, both meager.

At twenty-two, I was an earnest and tightly held together young woman, desperately focused on application to medical school. I think it peculiar (perhaps it is commonplace), but I often remember exactly where I was when a particular thought came to me—in the bathtub, driving a car, getting into an elevator. . . . Sometime the year I was twenty-two, I was holding a tray in line at a cafeteria in Cincinnati, Ohio, when I had the thought *There is something wrong with me because I do not know what I will do with my life if I don't get to go to medical school.* It wasn't just that I would be at a loss for what else to do; it was that I believed that my life somehow depended on it.

In a way, I was right. "One becomes a therapist because of his own desperation." That's what I heard four years later from Dr. Elvin Semrad, professor of psychiatry at Harvard Medical School, who in time became my mentor. It was through the process of becoming a psychiatrist and the practice of psychiatry—attending to the facts and feelings of my patients' lives while responsibly coming to know myself—that the formless despair of my childhood took shape and eventually faded, and my life opened to options I had never even dreamed of.

For sure, by the time I was thirty-five I had done a lot of living: as a child had been a prodigy on the piano; had, at fourteen, soloed with the Philadelphia Orchestra; had earned a full scholarship to Wellesley College; had married at twenty; had had a child while going to medical school; had divorced; had become a psychiatrist; had married and divorced again—but I didn't really begin to tap freely into my creative life until I was into my forties. In addition to what I learned from Semrad and from my personal psychoanalysis, the writings of a British pediatrician-become-psychiatrist had a profound impact on my coming to life. Dr. Donald W. Winnicott celebrated the muddle of the distinctly-not-perfect in whatever aspect of experience as the playground in which wholeness eventually may express itself. The stresses of my early life allowed in a steady haze—an apt description of the atmosphere, but not the memory, of my childhood. With all its cracks and crazing, this vessel holds.

On my fortieth birthday, in 1979, I visited Winnicott's widow, Claire, in her London home, where she hosted me for tea. Appreciating my regret that I had not had the opportunity to meet Dr. Winnicott while he lived (he had died in 1971), Mrs. Winnicott generously shared far more than her hospitality. She told me of a poignant note that Dr. Winnicott wrote to himself during his terminal illness:

Dear God, let me be alive when I die.

At sixty-five, I am grateful to be, in this sense, alive while I live.

In May 1995, I took a two-week break from my practice of psychiatry to complete the manuscript of *The Hormone of Desire*, a book about testosterone and women's health that I had researched for several years, was about half-written, and was due in a fortnight. Nine days of waking at first light to write all day and into the night, and it was done. On the tenth, the muse, apparently not yet ready to withdraw, woke me again at dawn to write something altogether other. I wrote some part of eight of these stories before the writing retreat came to its end.

A couple of years later, when my editor asked, "So what's your next book?" I remembered the urge of an earnest and naive twenty-two-year-old to write a grandiose and impossible book of wisdom and was grateful to be able actually to offer the beginnings of a book distilled from sixty years of conscious living and informed by a working lifetime of psychiatric practice. As life unfolded, the research and writing of yet another book intervened when, at the turn of the millennium, a potential crisis in women's health emerged in the form of a growing "anti-menstruation movement"—the proposal that women, even girls and young women, should, for the convenience of it, take hormones to do away with their periods. The essays and stories were on hold again until April 2003, when finally I sat to the challenge and pleasure of this writing.

The man who shot his toothbrush and the other clinical anecdotes I've used in this memoir made it through the fine filter for material protective of the relationships I have with my patients. In my view, termination of therapy should afford no exemption from this responsibility. I expected nothing less from the therapists to whom, at key times in my life, I turned for help. Notably, one of these gave me something more.

It happens when I am forty-eight and more than a dozen years past the end of a six-year Freudian analysis. I can say, in truth, that this work has given me my life, the most substantial of rewards. But it has also left me more *conscious*—of myself, of others, of the world—more tethered to *what's so* than I wish to be, and I long to have freer access to my imagination. When, near the end of my analysis, in 1974, I saw Peter Shaffer's play *Equus* on Broadway, I appreciated the concern written into the role of the psychiatrist, concern about the potential loss of a kind of intrinsic passion and freedom that might be the cost of reining in, through psychiatric analysis, the boy whose wildly out-of-control and violent actions require treatment. Subsequently I realized that the freedom I wished to have was a freedom that, in fact, I had never had. Before my analysis, I had watched myself and the world around me in an atmosphere of anxiety and despair. Now I watched myself and the world around me more comfortably. But still, I watched.

And so, a dozen or so years later, around 1986, I am attracted by an ad for a workshop in Cambridge to be given by Dr. Marian Woodman, a Jungian analyst from Toronto. What I know of Jung is limited to some vague sense that he was "wilder" than Freud, had dealt in archetypes (whatever they might be), and that he and Sigmund Freud had, around 1910, together traveled to the United States to give a series of lectures at Clark University in Worcester, the town where I grew up. Thus, virtually unencumbered by any significant knowledge of Jung, I approach Marian Woodman's workshop with curiosity and, on a much deeper level, with a wish that I might find some new way in to a stuck place in my psyche.

Dr. Woodman turns out to be charismatic, intelligent, eloquent, and, above all, alive. I am delighted, in particular, with this shared bit of her personal experience:

My analyst said to me: You will stand to your truth. You will do it kicking and screaming, or you will do it with grace, but you will do it.

Stand to your truth! Lord knows, I have tried—traditional psychotherapy, Freudian psychoanalysis, even some experience of psychodrama—and still I feel that some part of my most alive self remains closed off. *Could a Jungian analysis open this channel?*

Well, first I turn to books. I read Laurens van der Post's biography *Jung and the Story of Our Time,* and then Jung's memoir, transcribed from dictation: *Memories, Dreams, and Reflections.* I discover that Jung had had some unusual experiences exploring his own psyche. At one point, he spent considerable time in seclusion, immersed in what I understand to be waking dreams populated by extraordinary entities and symbols, inspired in his waking time to draw elaborate circular designs: mandalas. According to today's diagnostic criteria, this episode of Jung's life might have qualified as psychotic. But then, so would the visions that appeared to biblical figures and mystics. It's clear that the arena of spirituality is, in fact, a major point of difference between Jung and Freud.

My own exploration of the collective unconscious has been limited to the analyses of my dreams and those of my patients. Over the years, I have noticed that some dream elements seem to have meanings that carry through as common from person to person. For example, dreams of water or the ocean often seem to represent the person's psyche. Many of my patients report dreams that are variations on the theme of going down deep into water, dreams that in individual context bring the common understanding of anxiety about exploring thoughts and feelings in therapy. Another common dream symbol: women's wallets and handbags—which, as containers of valuables, often seem to represent the woman's womb. This interpretation was lent touching affirmation in the waking life of one of my patients when, during her convalescence from a hysterectomy, her mother came to visit her in the hospital carrying the gift of a capacious new pocketbook.

After several months of incubating the idea, finally I decide to consult with a Jungian analyst. I am hoping that a wider channel to my imagination and, possibly, to some spiritual connection to life itself may open, and that both my personal life and my work with patients will benefit. I expect that the experience will be, somehow, very different from the Freudian analysis I have had.

The mortal woman entrusted with this task has an office on Beacon Hill, around the corner and down the block from what will later become a Boston landmark, Cheers. Parking is a bitch. But her office is lovely and comfortable, complete with wood-burning fireplace. In sessions, while I talk, my Jungian analyst takes copious notes. I am disappointed, however, that she says very little. Since I am hoping that this work will stimulate some really juicy Jungian-type dreams, I'm frustrated when night after night yields nothing special to take to my sessions. After several weeks, I begin to feel that it is déjà vu all over again.

Preface

Consulting my journals today, I find the following entries:

November 07, 1987

    Had a session with C.D. that took me through a chronicle of the "Traumatic Experiences of My Infancy and Childhood"— Ugh, Ugh. She encouraged me to try to remember my dreams— (I couldn't recall a snatch this A.M.)—and then encouraged me not to try to help myself as a definitive healing, but to risk falling back a little and let the "Great Mother" come to me.

    I expect Kali.*

    God knows.

Well, finally I begin to dream, all right. I have nightmares like the worst of the darkest days of my Freudian analysis— stuff that I had been glad to let settle to the bottom and stay there. I have no appetite to stir it up again. I feel lousier and lousier. And there is no sign of the "Great Mother."

Just my Jungian analyst making her notes.

Then I have a dream unlike any I have had before, occurring as it does when I am in the space between sleeping and waking:

November 08, 1987

    I look through the mattress at the floor. The blue carpet is moving. Something breathing under it. A blue lipstick pokes through. ?penis. I get up to get M. [my lover]. A mask is propped up against the door. I see it move.

    Association: Ram Dass on LSD.

*Kali: the frightening Hindu goddess of destruction and creation.

This experience clinches it. Jung I am not. And neither is my analyst.

Before I quit the attempt, though, I get hung up over those notes the analyst has been making during our sessions. I find that I don't want to leave anything of myself with her except for her memories, and I ask if she will give the notes to me. Since they are not merely transcriptions of my dreams and associations but also contain her commentary, she is not comfortable about handing them over. She offers another solution, though: in our final session, she will burn them.

Transparent to both of us is the deeper meaning of the little drama we play out, as sheet by sheet she feeds the pages into her fireplace. Clearly the most healing aspect of my attempt to work with this gentle woman—and a powerfully healing experience it became for me—was her willingness to sacrifice something of hers in the service of respecting my need for privacy.

I have been scrupulous in what I have chosen to write in this memoir and grateful to the patients whose material does appear in these pages, included with the intention of presenting something of my most meaningful experiences as a psychiatrist, and not simply as a narrative of interesting clinical cases.

When I was a little girl, my maternal grandmother, in her Yiddish-English, used to say, *"Gay herein en nein heiser"*: "Go into nine houses . . . and you will see and hear the stuff of life to equal any fiction."

Here, at last, are my stories.

One

Becoming

*B*oundaries in the large extended family of my childhood were always something of a problem. Respect for separateness was not a birthright. Responsibility for self was not a hallmark. One of my cousins once said that she and her mother were "stuck together like a Popsicle." Epoxy resin is more like it. Popsicles at least melt.

Another sort of boundary had been stretched when my great-uncle married his niece. Think of it . . . my mother's oldest sister, Rose, married *her* mother's brother. My understanding is that they met when Rosie was ten or eleven or so and he was several years older and newly emigrated to America from

Russia, where all the family of that generation had been born. Eventually they fell in love, and they married.

My mother told me, with no comment and apparently no thought on the matter (though what she *really* thought about this and many another matter remained a mystery to me), "In the Jewish religion, an uncle can marry a niece, but an aunt can't marry a nephew." At the time, I thought that there was something odd, and maybe unfair, about this distinction.

I was a little girl who tended to think a lot, trying to figure out what was going on in my mother's head, in my family, and in the world around me. The Second World War figured large. Some decades later I put it together that the day I was born, Labor Day 1939, was just one day after Winston Churchill declared war on Germany. During my early childhood in Worcester, Massachusetts, the kitchen radio was always on with the war news about "the Allies" and a lot of other words I didn't understand, and with patriotic jingles encouraging us to buy war bonds.

> *Save up your pennies, and soon you'll have a nickel.*
> *Save up your nickels and soon you'll have a dime.*
> *We love our country, the stars make a banner*

("The stars make a banner . . ." that's how I sang it. I think now that those words probably were: *our star-spangled banner.*)

Soldiers and sailors in uniform were everywhere. Union Station was flooded with servicemen carrying lumpy duffel bags on their shoulders. In our neighborhood, the wail of air-raid sirens was a signal for the grown-ups to pull down the black window shades and turn off the lights. During one air-raid drill, my mother told me that she couldn't smoke her cigarette on the porch, because "the Germans might see the burning butt and know where to bomb us." Another time, in a bizarrely desperate effort to discourage me from eating what she considered junk food, she warned me off the State Line potato chips my Dad sold in his grocery store by telling me that "the Germans ground up glass in them." I wondered why my dad would sell them to anyone, and worried in particular about my friend Kathryn Rita Reilley, who ate those potato chips too. The war was a confusing, distant, and at the same time omnipresent element in my early life.

In clear contrast, that thing about Auntie Rosie being married to her uncle Bob seemed pretty natural. Their three kids, Dorothy (who I knew as Duchess), Noah (Sonny or Son), and Malcolm (Mally), were my favorite older cousins. When I was a little older, I figured out that Uncle Bob was both my uncle and my great-uncle, and of course I figured out that in addition to being their father, Uncle Bob was their great-uncle as well.

"Son" was short for "sunshine," the light his birth brought into the family soon after the sudden death of his maternal grandfather Noah, for whom he was named. I never even wondered how Duchess got her name. I was two or three when we moved in with the family for a while, and Duchess was twenty—tall, beautiful in an exotic sort of way, and with an alluring mole on her cheek, like Elizabeth Taylor. I remember standing at the bathroom door, watching her dress her hair—puffing a pompadour secured by curved hair combs above her forehead, and, at the sides and the back, pinning the ends over a U-shaped loop of sausagelike padding called a "rat," this part of the hairdo secured by a fancy, decorated string hairnet. Rodent metaphors extended to the rat-tailed comb, whose skinny end she used to tuck the hair around the "rat." My straight, thick brown hair was in a Dutch clip, sort of like what Hans Brinker might have worn, and I was mesmerized by Duchess's coiffure—rat and all.

At that time, my cousin Son was sixteen, and Mally a couple of years younger. Once in a while the two of them would get into some horseplay, with which Auntie Rosie didn't have much patience. She'd chase them around the house, flailing ineffectually with Uncle Bob's belt and yelling for them to quit it. I loved the excitement. Having a little girl in the house for a couple of months must have been more of a novelty than a nuisance for them, as they were very kind to me. Imagine my sixteen-year-old boy cousin creating magical adventures for me in a large clump of lilac bushes in the backyard, where he pushed aside the branches with their shiny green heart-shaped leaves and cautioned me to step carefully over the gnarled roots, whispering for me to watch for the gremlins who lived there. Although they never actually made an appearance, I knew exactly what they looked like.

Years later I realized that my parents weren't much older than Duchess or Son. Auntie Rosie was the second oldest of eight children, my mother the youngest and only nine when Duchess was born. Those nine years did seem to constitute a generation, though. I always felt that Duchess was much like an older sister to me.

My mother had met my dad in Springfield, Massachusetts,

in 1937 or so, when she was working as a traveling demonstrator for Sears and Roebuck (a notably independent job for a woman in those days) and he was managing something I heard as "growerzoutlet," which must have been a produce market. I knew my dad's workplace had something to do with food, but I never knew exactly what it was or imagined how its name might be spelled.

Virtually a hush-hush family secret: not until they went to take out a marriage license did my mother learn that her prospective husband was *nearly two years younger* than she—born in 1915 to her 1913. This small difference in age, compounded by the dissembling, became a condensing point for the atmosphere of disappointment and distrust that had, perhaps since her father dropped dead of a heart attack when she was twelve, clouded my mother's experience of life.

My parents began married life in Springfield, where I was born and where we lived until I was about two. Then my father was offered a job in Connecticut. This was trouble, since the tacit limit of acceptable distance from Worcester and my mother's family had been Springfield. The family pull—that we move not farther away but back to Worcester—prevailed.

Memory, for me, begins at this point, in Worcester at my grandmother's house, when we moved in with her and my aunt, uncle, and cousins—all nine of us sharing the top-floor apartment in the three-decker on Houghton Street. My parents slept on the couch in the living room, I think that my crib was in the dining room, and I know that a cardboard carton full of my toys and books was in the boys' room. The sides of that box came up to my armpits, and I remember the sharpness of the box edge on my upper chest when I leaned over into it to reach my Betsy Wetsy.

The dominant presence in the household, such that Auntie Rosie, Uncle Bob, and their kids were said to be living with her rather than the other way around, was my grandmother, Bobba. Never mind that Uncle Bob paid the rent; it was always "Bobba's house." Enclaves of extended family lived or worked nearby. A few blocks away in different directions were Bobba's two sisters, Boonie and Tanteh, with their families, and one of her brothers, Uncle Ike, owned the corner grocery store where my mother bought cigarettes and where I could get an ice cream.

Auntie Rosie didn't buy much food at Uncle Ike's, though. She and my mother shopped at the Jewish kosher markets on Water Street. I loved to go with them. All that hustle and bustle, sound, color, and smells. "The chickenik," Josephs' chicken store, had live chickens in doweled crates stacked up against the wall. The men behind the counter wore hats—skullcaps or fedoras, sometimes with the front brim pushed up, the better to see. Josephs' stank of burned chicken feathers. I used to pass the time waiting for our turn making designs with my shoe in the sawdust scattered on the floor to collect dirt and spills.

Pulda's kosher fish market sold only fish with scales, of course—no shrimp, lobster, clams, or catfish—and was a different kind of stinky. Sometimes we would skip Cohen's kosher meat market, because they delivered. I remember my mother on the telephone: "Mitzi, I want a good brisket. Not a double, a single." On Water Street, we always shopped at Whitman's creamery, where the lox was sliced only by hand, and where my aunt bought farmer cheese, "a nice whitefish," groceries, and a block of halvah. Smoked fish, but no other stinky smells here. And then: Weintraub's Delicatessen. My mouth waters remembering the aromas and flavors there: hot pastrami, corned beef, pickled tongue, half-sour pickles, and sour green tomatoes. Palisades of salamis hung above the men behind the counter spooning mustard into cones of brown waxed paper to accompany whatever we bought to go. Our last stop might be Lieberman's Bakery—fragrant with pumpernickel and cornmeal-dusted rye breads, and with cases of babke, *kichel*, nut-studded mandel bread, half-moon cookies, cakes and pastries, and trays of chocolate éclairs and charlotte russes.

Indeed much of life centered around food, its purchase, its preparation, and its consumption. For Shabbas (the Sabbath), Bobba always baked one or another cake and, always, challah. Every Friday, I would find the huge golden ceramic mixing bowl covered with a dish towel over the bread dough rising, then Bobba in her housedress and bibbed print apron standing at the kitchen table, dashing flour at the wooden bread board. I loved to watch as she cut off a hunk of challah dough, pressed it down with the heel of her hand, and folded it quickly over to press again and again. She usually gave me my own little mound of dough to knead. By the time I was through with it, my challie didn't look much like hers, but she painted it carefully with egg yolk and baked it anyway. My dolls didn't mind that it had the texture of a rock and looked like one, for that matter.

To crown her beautiful challahs, Bobba usually made braids

of dough—the shape of the challah and the placement of the braid determined by proximity to holidays. I never learned the code. Sometimes the challah was round, with a braid encircled like a wreath, but most times the challah was oval, and the braid lay centered on top in a straight line lengthwise. When my grandmother took the bread out of the oven to cool, she would denude one of the challahs of its braid and give it to me hot, to eat, with butter. I have never had its equal.

For Shabbas, Auntie Rosie usually made gefilte fish, grinding the fish in a hand grinder that screwed onto the top of the kitchen table: a piece of raw fish into the mouth of the grinder, a piece of onion to push the fish down, a hand clamped over the top of the grinder to hold it all in place, fish and onion juice dripping. Messy work that made her eyes tear up, and there was no helping the ground fish lost to coating the fish grinder.

I was born with a taste for Jewish-Russian food and always enjoyed the poached fish balls decorated with carrot and served with beet-juice-colored horseradish. I liked to eat them hot in their poaching broth. I make gefilte fish today pretty much as my aunt and my mother did—but with the convenience of raw fish ground to order by the fish market and onions ground in a blender jar. I know it's not rational, but I have held the line against owning a food processor—one less technological advance removed from the hand grinder of my childhood.

Cooking with Bobba wasn't the only activity we shared. Sometimes she and I (on her lap) sat by the window counting cars. Most of them were black. When traffic was light, she taught me Russian songs: *Cheesik, cheesik, justin bil, Oofcantoro vodkoo pil*. (Bird, bird, where are you? I'm with the cantor, drinking vodka!)

Sometimes she let me take the hairpins out of the bun at the back of her head and comb her long, silky white hair with a big wide-toothed comb. I tried each time to do the bun up again, but never could get it to stay. Finally Bobba would twist her hair and pin it back up deftly with those hands I will never forget.

Bobba's hands were very soft, as was, physically, everything about her. Her cheeks were soft, her breasts were soft, and her belly, into which I leaned when I was finished on the toilet and she came in to wipe me, was soft. I remember my head in her apron, looking down at Bobba's shoes—black, with laces and eyelet cutouts—while she wadded up the toilet paper and wiped me clean. It felt different from when my mother did it. Softer.

We lived at Bobba's house for several months, until my father found a job managing the dairy department of Brockelman's, a food emporium on Main Street. Last time I looked, the building was still there, vacant and proud, with the frieze of produce and upside-down chickens on the columns that mark its corners. Once my dad was set with work, my mother, my father, and I moved to an apartment on the other side of town, and then in the sixteen years before I went to college, we moved six times. Bobba and retinue moved only once, and Bobba's house was a steady, warm, and flavorful center to it all.

My mother's seven older sibs included five brothers. Fatherless from age twelve, she was especially attached to them—even (and particularly) to the one, Barney, who taught me the meaning of "black sheep." I was told he was charming—he had no difficulty in attracting wives—but I did not find him so.

Particularly unwelcome were the times at Bobba's house when the family might be gathered for shabbas dinner or . . . come to think of it, there was nearly always some constellation of people eating, or having tea or coffee, or playing pinochle with those decks of cards that were missing a lot of numbers. Anyway, in the midst of a pleasant time, the phone would ring, someone would answer, and everything would change. It was Barney calling. Gambling. He needed money again. "They'll break his knees if he doesn't pay."

His three sisters, Auntie Rosie, Auntie Bess, and my mother, would find some way to scrape together the money and *sendittohimWesternUnion*. I wondered why Barney never called on his brothers for help. Maybe he did. Maybe they had the guts to say no.

At intervals for years, tension and raised voices came from my parents' bedroom after the Barney calls. By the time I was five, my dad was working dawn to dark in his own grocery store six days a week, and the profit margin was small. Robert's Market, where my dad did all the work, from cutting meat to making window-display signs for the weekly specials, was in a neighborhood of families whose breadwinners worked in the wire mill down the hill, a factory that regularly laid people off. My dad carried them for months, scribbling names onto curling bits of cash register receipts that he put into a little wooden file box, hopefully to be tallied up and paid when the customer was called back to work and able. Dad never refused credit, and he was not always paid.

One day when I was about five, Barney showed up with a lovely blond wife called Chaddy—short for Charlotte. I overheard my mother say that Chaddy, whose family lived in some faraway place called Portland, Oregon, was *a blueblood* and was listed in the New York Social Register. My mother had a copy of the blue book to prove it. Chaddy's family owned property in many states, including, as fate would have it, a home and a vacant store in Auburn, a suburb of Worcester. Barney decided to become a grocer. Oh boy.

During the next few years, Barney and Chaddy had two babies; Barney sold groceries, took the cash from the till, and bet on the horses. One day, Chaddy took her baby girls to Oregon to visit her family and did not come back. Then Barney went out there to get them and could not find them.

I remember one very scary night when, after I went to bed, I heard high-pitched wailing coming from the living room, where Barney was crying about his family. My mother thought up a plan of writing a letter to Walter Winchell, whose radio show we listened to every Sunday night. That broadcast began with the sound of a teletype key: *beep beep da beep beep, beep beep da beep beep . . . Good evening, Mr. and Mrs. North America and all the ships at sea, let's go to press . . .* But Mother's was an idea before its time. *Unsolved Mysteries* was not Winchell's focus.

The plan devolved to trying to hire a detective to look for Chaddy and the girls. Money was, of course, a problem. For two years, since kindergarten (*Save up your pennies, and soon you'll have a nickel. / Save up your nickels and soon you'll have a* dime. / *We love our country, the stars make a banner . . .*), I had brought a quarter to school each week to buy war stamps, and by second grade, I had enough stamps to qualify for the shiny white cardboard certificate with illustrations of Snow White and the Seven Dwarfs and Thumper all around the border, and with some official-looking writing and a gold sticker at the bottom—a twenty-five-dollar war bond. My parents had ceremoniously put the certificate in the small gray metal box with a lock—the "strong box"—in which they kept important papers. The morning after the night of the crying, my mother told me that I had to give my bond to Barney. I refused, but they made me give it to him anyway.

I never saw Chaddy or the children again. A few snapshots of the babies and a set of Tiffany demitasse cups are the only traces that remain. I never worried about the girls. They were with their mother, whom I liked a lot, and I knew that Barney was trouble. Still, for years and years I felt guilty when I remembered refusing to offer Barney my bond. Decades later, when I learned that "guilt is sometimes just guilt, but sometimes it's resentment turned inside out," I recognized my anger for what it was and could finally extend compassion to myself and, eventually, to the grown-ups who couldn't do any better.

Back at that dark time in my early childhood, Barney declared bankruptcy, left his suppliers holding the bag, and left town. I would have been glad never to see him again, but he was destined to turn up at a nodal point, five years later, when I was twelve.

While my mother had been unwell in one way or another

for as long as I could remember, when I was twelve her health began seriously to degenerate. At one point I remember thinking that not a single part of her body worked without some problem. She was in the hospital, very sick after gall bladder surgery, when I had my first menstrual period. That's when Barney showed up with another wife, this time a feisty brown-haired Irishwoman named Dot.

The events fuse together for me: my passage to womanhood, my mother sick in the hospital, and Barney with his new wife sleeping on the couch in our living room. Alone with a tangle of feelings I couldn't sort out, I did not know that the seeds of my eventual choice of profession had been sown.

I became a physician in part out of the wish to heal my mother.

I became a psychiatrist for certain out of the need to heal myself.

Two

Mother, Music, and Me

L*ikely a close second to the formative and deformative in-*fluence of her father's death when she was twelve was my mother's having grown up in the shadow of her two-year-older brother, Harry, who was a child prodigy on the violin. My mother used to tell with pride that when her father was alive, every one of the eight children was given music lessons. Early on, Harry showed such musical gifts that he was brought to the attention of a Worcester patron, Mrs. Homagage (Mrs. Homer Gage, I later figured out), who sponsored his study in New York City with Leopold Hour (Auer, ditto). Quite recently I discovered that my uncle had been taught by the great

Hungarian violinist, whose pupils had included Mischa Elman and Jascha Heifetz.

As though she had been there herself, my mother spoke about her brother Harry's first meeting, when he was still a young boy, with Leopold Auer. As she told it, Mr. Auer was, at that time, very old, virtually blind, and reluctant to take a new student. Having been importuned at least to hear Harry play, during the audition the maestro approached Harry, felt the positions of his arms, and roughly adjusted them. *Hold your arm up! Keep your elbow in!* Then, he felt Harry's smooth face. *But you're only a boy!* And so it was that he took Harry on as a pupil.

From newspaper clippings, I learned that, following his debut, Harry toured European musical centers and then returned to play Carnegie Hall as the kickoff of an American tour. I remember a creased black-and-white photo that my mother carried in her wallet of a foreign-language theatre billboard with the name Melnikoff printed large and with Harry wearing a caped coat and standing in the foreground.

Those were harrowing economic times—1929 to 1930—the first years of the Depression that slammed the nation and compounded difficulties for my mother's family five years into life without her father. I have painful imaginings of the family straining to scrape together resources for the trip to New York to hear Harry play at Carnegie Hall. Whatever the circumstances, I can hardly understand how it was that my mother, who was seventeen years old at the time, could have been left behind while the rest of the family attended the concert. As "consolation," she was brought back some dessert treat—

a pitiful detail she told with muted (and understandable) bitterness.

When I was a little girl and first knew him, my uncle Harry was a successful professional musician, married, and living in Riverdale, New York. He was a contractor for RCA recordings and played in Vaughn Monroe's and Perry Como's orchestras. Checking a discography, I find listings of Harry Melnikoff on dozens of recordings with popular artists of the 1940s, '50s, and '60s, including Harry Belafonte, Frankie Laine, Tito Puente, The Weavers, Eartha Kitt, Chris Connor, and Charlie Parker (*Charlie Parker with Strings*).

As a kid, I used to watch *The Perry Como Show* on TV for the moment when the camera panned the orchestra, and I could easily pick out my uncle Harry by the white handkerchief he draped between the fiddle and his chin. Once, sometime in the 1950s, Vaughn Monroe was featured at the Meadows—a night-club he owned that was a glamorous spot for dinner dancing in Framingham, not far from Worcester. It wasn't Carnegie Hall, but my mother proudly took me to a rehearsal, where my uncle introduced me to the singer, whose autographed picture is taped in a dusty album with the archives of my own musical life.

That began when I was four—when I discovered the old upright piano at Bobba's house. Mice had nested in the strings, with interesting consequences. Not all of the keys would play. When I began picking out tunes on the keyboard, my mother must have been excited at the possibility that she had hatched a next-generation wunderkind. Certainly she lost no time in arranging for me to have piano lessons. No way was this little girl of hers going to be left behind. The purchase of a new

Emerson spinet piano took priority by several years over the acquisition of our first family car.

My first piano teacher, Madeleine Sadick, was a beautiful, graceful, dark-eyed young woman who reminded me of a princess in my books of fairy tales. I remember the elegant evening dresses hanging behind her studio door in the building up the steep hill from Steinert's music store on Main Street. I imagined that she wore one or another of them when her prince came to take her to the ball. I may have been close to correct in this.

Madeleine began by teaching me to close my fingers over my curled thumb, place my little hand on middle C, and allow it to open "like a snail," keeping my fingers curled as I played. I learned to read music before I could read words, but from the first, I found it easier to listen to a piece of music and play it back by ear than to read the score.

From the time I was four, a high point of going downtown every Saturday morning for piano lessons was lunch at Easton's, a soda fountain on Main Street that also sold tobacco and magazines. For lunch, violating several laws of kashruth simultaneously, I usually had a BLT with a chocolate frappe. Come to think of it, I'm not sure that drinking milk while eating bacon qualifies as a double whammy. To quote one of my dad's aphorisms: "Once you're wet, you're wet."

When I was old enough to be wild for comic books, most times at Easton's my mother treated me to *five* ten-cent issues—Wonder Woman (*Holy Hera, protect me!*) my favorite. Lunch was often followed by a visit to Ephraim's toy store. My primary interest there was the book section, the source of my collection first of green-bound Bobbsey Twins adventures and later of blue-bound Nancy Drew mysteries. After Ephraim's, we might make a stop at Denholm's department store, which had a lending library, where, for a penny or two a day, my mother borrowed the newest popular novels covered in cellophane. Finally, we'd visit the downtown branch of the Worcester Public Library—the children's room for me, and the grown-up library for my mother, who was a reader with tastes running to historical and romantic novels.

At home, my mother usually had a couple of books stacked on the floor beside her chair in the living room. Without a doubt, her own interest in reading and her support for my passion for books occasioned the best-feeling experiences we ever shared. My mother's dramatic intonation of the title of one of her favorites, *The Sun Is My Undoing*, stands out as an audible memory. I never knew, but I wanted to, what moved her about this book. Our shared experiences were limited to transacting the business of finding books to read, and did not extend to discussing them.

I remember the day I was first allowed, at age twelve or so, a library card for limited access to the adult library. Room after room of shelved grown-up books offered an overwhelming choice. I ventured as far as the B's and, recognizing some books I had known my mother to read, I began with the works of Pearl Buck. Week after week, I read my way through in alphabetical order of title, until I had read them all. At that point, it seemed like a good idea simply to read the next volume on the shelf. This turned out to be a book by Lillian Budd called *April Snow*. Taking its title from Scandinavian lore—*snow in April means a fertile season*—it was a novel about a beleaguered Scandinavian woman whose husband kept her barefoot in winter and pregnant in summer. As the tale unfolded, each year it snowed, and each year the exhausted woman had another baby. At twelve, I found the story scary and depressing, and I was afraid to choose another book on that shelf. In fact, I believe that I didn't read another book in the adult library at all for a while. Like most of the confusing and difficult experiences of my young life, I was alone with this.

My mother must have read books to me before I could read, but I have no clear memory of it. I can't remember sitting on her lap. The saddest fact is that I don't remember her touching me with affection, ever. I remember her saying that, when I was an infant, she used to massage me with baby oil after my bath. I think she said that I loved it. I like to think that. I know she said that when she was finished, I looked like a Greek olive. By the time I was three and came to memory, though, the touching was only functional. I remember, on winter days, standing naked on a chair by the kitchen sink (the kitchen being the warmest room in the flat) while my mother washed and dried me, limb by limb. Her touch in this, as when she brushed my hair, was businesslike, to get the job done.

I remember too, on school nights, after I went to bed, listening to the creak and thump of the ironing board being opened and stood upright, followed by the swishing sounds of my mother ironing one of my smocked, sashed dresses (from Best & Company, ordered from the catalog and costing more than we could really afford). It was a point of pride with her to send me to school each day wearing a freshly pressed dress.

I lay in my bed at night, listening, and wishing that I were the dress, my mother's hands upon *me*, touching me with love and care.

One extraordinary weekday morning when I was seven or so, my parents kept me home from school for the treat of going downtown with my dad while my mother minded the store. Happy to be with him, I remember being puzzled when he took me past Ephraim's Toys, around the corner, and into an unfamiliar office building, then up an elevator to approach a door on whose opaque glass I made out the words

DR. MAYCOCK
Exodontist

On that miserable day in my childhood, worse than the trauma of being forced into the dentist's chair, held down, given gas, and waking with two teeth missing and a bloody mouth, was my dad's having betrayed my trust. Even more painful and more enduringly consequential than the betrayal was my being awakened to powerful anger at the parent for whom I had heretofore known only love. I remember my terrified, helpless rage in the dentist's office, a little girl of seven standing lonely and small next to the chair, when I summoned up the worst thing I could think to scream at my father:

You son-of-a-bitch!

Neither he nor I understood the depth of pain and loss I suffered that day. When I was old enough to manage the perspective, I came, of course, to forgive my father for not hav-ing prepared me for something disagreeable that had to be done ultimately for my benefit. But I have spent a lifetime try-ing to avoid circumstances that might refuel the fire of helpless rage ignited in me that sad day.

I can't imagine how my life would have turned out had I not had the comfort in my growing-up years of the times I spent in the company of my mother's next-older sister, my aunt Bess, together with her husband, Al, and their two sons, Neal and Fred. When I was about ten, their family moved to Worcester from Atlanta when Uncle Al was transferred *for a very important job*—to take over as manager of the Worcester division of the United States Envelope Company.

As a consequence of the postwar housing shortage, Aunt Bess, Uncle Al, Neal, and Fred were accommodated for the first several months in a suite of rooms at Worcester's grand downtown hotel, the Sheraton. When a vacancy at Salisbury Gardens (not far from Worcester Tech, where Uncle Al had gone to college) finally opened up, they moved into a two-story garden apartment that was, to me, exotic and luxurious. Auntie Bess and Uncle Al frequently welcomed my little-girl presence, invited me often to dinner, and included me in an occasional Sunday family trip to Boston to see the circus or the rodeo at Boston Garden. The sweetest times of my life be-came the couple of weeks' vacation I spent with them each year at Cape Cod, where I could relax in the gentle affection that was the atmosphere of the surround—a life-giving break from the tension and coldness of my home.

* * *

I never understood why learning to play piano came easily to me. Truly, I didn't practice very much. I remember seeing other, even older kids sitting stiffly at the keyboard, straining to get their fingers to play the notes. From the beginning, I was dexterous, and I swayed into the music as I played. At yearly recitals and in national competitions, I was a young star—but as time passed, my heart was clearly elsewhere. The truth was, I would rather have been dancing.

When I was nine, I saw the movie *The Red Shoes*, with Moira Shearer. The darkness of the Svengali theme was eclipsed for me by the grace and movement of the ballet dancer, twirling on her toes, floating in ethereal costumes. I begged for ballet lessons. The impediment was more than financial. I was a skinny little girl, and stood next to the smallest, Lois Gold, when we lined up by height at school. Although basically healthy, when I was six I'd had an attack of acute appendicitis and a midnight appendectomy—one of the most terrifying experiences of my life. Nobody had told me anything like the truth about what was happening. Since I had had the usual childhood warnings against putting things over my head or mouth because of the danger of suffocation, when the ether mask was clamped to my face, I thought I was being killed. Choking on the fumes, I screamed, "Take it off! Take it off! I'll be a good girl! I'll be a good girl."

What I know about my infancy goes a distance to account for the cautious, frightened look in the eyes that projects from the photographs of my childhood. "Colic" was what they said explained my having screamed for the first three months of my life. Apparently I hardly slept, so nobody else did either. My mother's friend Bette was even called in for reinforcements. I was told that the only thing that stopped my screaming was being held and "walked the floor." My father once demonstrated his method of quieting me—swinging me in his arms vigorously from side to side. I wonder whether this was comforting so much as that it took my breath away.

One time during the exhausting first few months of my infancy, when finally I fell asleep, my mother noticed that I had wet my diaper. Fearing that I would wake up if she changed me yet determined that I be dry, she decided to cut away the wet diaper with a scissors. When my father saw her approaching me with shears in hand, fearing that her intention was the unspeakable, he screamed out her name to stop her.

Through my growing-up years, this incident was regularly recounted with amusement, regardless of my presence and oblivious to the fact that I still experienced myself to be *too much* for my parents in one way or another. I never found the story funny.

Another event with disturbing resonance was something that ensued when my mother decided to wean me from the bottle before I was a year old. She came up with the idea of demonstrating to me that the bottles and nipples were "all gone" by cutting up the nipples with a scissors before my eyes. (Ugh! What could have possessed her to do such a thing?) It seems that I was an early talker. If it is to be believed, I spoke sentences and sang songs at nine months. As the story went on: a day or so later, she was wheeling me in a carriage past a drugstore where there was a window display of baby bottles.

I am said to have pointed and screamed out, "There they are!"—while my mother raced us past the window.

Of course, I have no memory of these events. I do remember, from the time I was six, my mother's dramatic recounting of the details of my emergency appendectomy. Out of touch with my experience and focused on hers, as was her way, she reported: *Just as the surgeon removed the appendix, it burst in his hands.* In then-recent pre-antibiotic times, peritonitis was often lethal.

This apparently close call reinforced my mother's basic attitude of hovering and intrusive concern. Regularly she dosed me with miserable-tasting thick "tonics" and disgusting mineral oil, insisted that to stay warm from October to May I wear long cotton stockings safety-pinned to tabs on my undershirts, and layered on the clothes. Encased in a snowsuit, I remember sucking in my little belly and feeling the sweaters and snowsuit around me like a shell that could have stood on its own.

At nine I wanted so much to dance that I did not quit importuning for ballet until, finally, my mother relented and signed me up. Oh, the excitement of buying the black leotard, tights, and Capezio ballet slippers with elastic to be sewn across the instep and with strings to pull tight around my foot. I loved ballet class. The bar exercises: *first, second, third positions; plié; reach down, up . . .*

Holding on to the back of a kitchen chair, I practiced at home every chance I could. Before long, my mother became frantic and began haranguing me to stop. *You'll make yourself sick with this dancing. You're too skinny for all that exercise.* After a few weeks, she simply refused to take me to class. I was devastated.

Thinking about it still gives me a bad feeling in my chest. For years, I squeezed my toes into those flat ballet slippers and tried to stand on point in them, dreaming about being a dancer.

Of course, there was no question but that I continue to study piano. Sadly, except for the beginning, when I picked out tunes on Bobba's old upright, playing piano was not "mine." It seemed that everyone else—most particularly, my mother— took more pleasure in my playing than I did. For years, her involvement in my musical experience was total. She sat through every piano lesson and every daily practice session.

I would have done better with less.

If I could have spoken my mind at eight, when my lovely piano teacher, Madeleine, passed me on to *her* teacher, Marie Louise Webb-Betts, I would have resisted. But my mother was thrilled at the evidence of my musical mastery, and dutifully I went along.

Mrs. Betts was a middle-aged matron by no means willowy, with no hint of a ball gown on any door, and with two grand pianos in her parlor. She belonged to an organization called The National Guild of Piano Teachers, and every spring her select pupils prepared for competition, where we demonstrated our technical skills to visiting judges: scales and arpeggios played from bass to middle C; hands dividing, right hand climbing up to treble and left simultaneously roaring down to bass; hands coming back together to middle C and returning together to bass. Then we played pieces chosen from a specified repertoire that included Bach inventions, preludes, and fugues, Mozart sonatas, and, ultimately, concertos. Each spring, too, Mrs. Betts's living room was transformed into a recording studio to provide the means for long-distance judging. I still have a couple of crackly 78s of "Rustling of Spring" and of a Tchaikovsky piano concerto I played, warping away in my collection.

Another annual happening: each fall, Worcester hosted its main cultural event: the Music Festival. Those years, the Philadelphia Orchestra under the direction of Eugene Ormandy and William Smith came to perform a full week of concerts in the Worcester Municipal Auditorium at Lincoln Square. For the month leading up to the gala, the downtown department stores and women's dress shops featured window displays with a musical theme and with mannequins in evening gowns. For many years my older cousin Duchess took me to the Saturday morning children's concerts. When I was fourteen, and recommended as qualified for the opportunity by my junior high school music teacher, Miss Lynch, I was invited to be a soloist.

Appropriate for the Concert for Young People, the piece I was to play was Tchaikovsky's "Dance of the Sugarplum Fairy" from the *Nutcracker Suite*. The part called for a celeste—an instrument similar to a piano but with a shorter keyboard and strings that yield bell-like tones. In the early summer, well in advance of the October concert, a crated instrument arrived at my home from Philadelphia. I studied and practiced the score of that little piece note by note—no way to chance playing by ear on this occasion.

As the time grew close, what good feeling I had about performing with the orchestra was muted when my dad told me that he wouldn't be able to be there. *I can't afford to close on a Saturday morning.* In 1953 small grocers were having a hard time competing for business with the new "super" markets. Shades of Carnegie Hall 1930, but this time it was I who was sadly disappointed.

The day of the concert: there I was in my three-quarter-sleeved, full-skirted red taffeta dress. Mrs. Eugene Ormandy sat with me backstage, assuring me that jitters were a universal phenomenon. I recall that she said something about the green room getting its name "because performers turn green there." Before I played, the conductor invited me to the microphone for a few words. I don't remember what I said. Thankfully, I played my piece without a hitch. After the concert, kids came backstage for me to autograph their programs. The experience felt something like a dream.

Vivid to me, in contrast, was my father's showing up backstage after it was all over, excitedly proclaiming that of course he was there for the performance and how could he possibly have missed it? No matter that it would have meant something different to me to have known he would be there in the audience, and that his experience of not missing something was not mine. In later years, he would sometimes make proud reference to my "illustrious childhood," which he had chronicled in a display he made with clippings of my accomplishments and propped on the shelf behind the checkout counter of Robert's Market, next to the cigarettes. I didn't like to look at them. Nobody recognized how unseen I was and how lonely and lost I felt.

After the music festival, the Worcester papers made much

of their local girl's performance with the Philadelphia Orchestra. There, on the front page of the *Worcester Telegram and Gazette,* was my photo with a review of the concert and the notation that I had played "with impeccable accuracy and polished style." Someone contacted my teacher with the proposal that I play a concerto with the orchestra when I was ready. I dreaded that prospect. "The Dance of the Sugarplum Fairy" had not been much of a technical challenge, but I did not want to take on the work of practicing enough to trust my hands in performance of a substantially more demanding piece. At fourteen, though, I was not yet ready to resist the tide, and when Mrs. Betts urged that I move on to study in Boston and arranged an audition for me with Heinrich Gebhard (who had been Leonard Bernstein's piano teacher), I went along.

I didn't know enough to be awed by Gebhard. I had all I could do to understand his heavily accented English and to deal with his attempt to change my piano technique. The latter was, in particular, Not a Good Thing.

Since age four, I had been taught a way of playing piano that was, by this time, second nature to me. Watching concert artists, I had observed more than one approach to playing the piano. I had noticed that some of them kept their wrists high, while I was disciplined to keep mine low and steady; some pianists used their fingers like hammers, lifting them high off the keys, while I had been taught to keep my fingers on the keys and to press rather than strike them. After I struggled through several frustrating lessons with Gebhard, my mother consulted Mrs. Betts, who defended the technique she had taught: "the latter method of Theodor Leschetizky." This mouthful of a name stayed in my brain, and Leschetizky's technique stayed in my body. Gebhard might as well have tried to get me to write left-handed. I remember actually feeling nauseous when I tried to follow his direction. I was very much relieved when arrangements were made for me to study, instead, with Jules Wolffers, professor of music at Boston University, who had no bone to pick with Leschetizky. Beginning when I was fifteen, my mother drove us to Wolffers's home in Waban, a suburb west of Boston, for weekly piano lessons.

I've been told that my uncle Harry had urged, early on, to have me study harp, since harpists (unlike pianists) were in short supply for the major orchestras, and he had the practical idea that, as a harpist, I would be assured a secure musical career. No matter that even as a child, in the way children speak about such things, I had never said that I wanted to be a musician when I grew up. I had never even thought it.

I remember my last piano teacher, Jules Wolffers, as compatible and really very patient, even while, as I began to come into my own, I practiced less and less. When, at sixteen, I began to date, the doors to a life beyond my family began to open, and I was drawn to new possibilities like dammed water freed to flow out to the sea. I didn't have much of a sense of self, I didn't have much of a sense of others, the world of adults was oceanic, and I felt very small, but I carried with me one life-directing, in many (but not all) ways, valuable legacy of my childhood: the belief that, if I tried, there was nothing I could not accomplish.

That year, 1955, I was a junior at Classical High School

when I met a nineteen-year-old sophomore at Clark University who, like my piano teacher, was also named Jules. "Julie" Rako had been born in Belgium. In the early 1940s his family had, like other European Jews who had found a way to do so, fled the Nazi occupation. Julie lived in Cuba until he was about nine, and subsequently grew up in New York City. French had been his first language, although he had never learned to read or write it. He spoke perfect English, was fluent in Spanish, had intense dark eyes, and seemed to me altogether exotic. He also had a grey Ford Fairlane. Before long, Julie began to take over from my mother the task of driving me to Boston for my piano lessons. We drove to Boston other times, too—for dancing at the Totem Pole Ballroom at Norumbega Park, for dinner at the pagoda of Chin's Village in Wellesley, or to Polynesian Village at the Somerset Hotel. Delicious times. Warm times. I discovered that it felt wonderful to be touched. The piano just faded away.

Resistance from my mother to (in her view) my giving up a concert career was notably (and blessedly) absent—an expression, I'm afraid, more of her chronic depressive resignation— *Woe is me. It's my fate to be disappointed. Nothing ever works out the way I wish*—than of her willingness to accept my choice with grace. Another element that influenced her laissez-faire (and provided a substitute focus) was my having decided to be a doctor. There could have been no more acceptable next best thing. Never mind that I was only sixteen; the fact that my boyfriend was premed as well completed her picture of a desirable future for me.

*   *   *

I did not play the piano at all for seventeen full and bumpy years into that future. Several years into a personal psycho-analysis, I found myself wanting to try the piano once again—this time on my own terms. I thought I might perhaps find pleasure in playing chamber music. Certainly I did not need so grand a teacher, but fate had it that I found my way to Wolfe Wolfinsohn, violinist and retired leader of the Stradivarius String Quartet. Wolfinsohn introduced me to a neophyte cellist, a young woman named Allie, and generously offered to coach us both.

I had my work cut out for me. Piano parts in chamber pieces are challenging, and I hadn't practiced for a very long time. Quite soon I began clearly to take more pleasure in a newly stimulated interest in listening to recordings of Casals than in playing, either alone or with Allie. For one thing, when she and I practiced together, very often Allie's tone was disturbingly sharp or flat. I was so green that I thought that her cello was simply out of tune, and I would ask her repeatedly to adjust its tuning. I didn't realize that the intonation was in this instance a function of her finger placement, and of course tuning the instrument again and again did not solve the problem.

After several months, there came a day, miserere, when Wolfie was pleased enough with the Brahms sonata to suggest that we perform a musicale. He proposed, graciously, that he and his wife, Sally, host the little event in the drawing room of their lovely home on Hilliard Street in Cambridge. I came to wish that I had quashed the idea from the start. Oh, Allie and

I played well enough to our appreciative audience of friends and family, but the music we made was not, to me, beautiful. I knew that I'd have to work a lot harder than I was willing in order to play well enough to suit myself and to carry my part with more experienced and skilled musicians. Ultimately, I was unable to open a channel of joy for myself in playing piano, and I gave up the effort once again.

Sometime in the late 1980s, in the company of an intimate friend who was both a psychiatrist and a Buddhist, I attended a conference in New York entitled "Buddhism and Psychotherapy." He and I took a workshop taught by John Daido Loori, Sensei, a former sailor who had left the sea to study Buddhism and to become guru of a Buddhist monastery in upstate New York. Abbott Loori offered the observation, with regard to reincarnation, that *we live several lives in each lifetime*. I say amen to that.

Music in my present lifetime? I enjoy an occasional concert, but mostly I listen to recorded music—more often and with more pleasure than ever. I play piano for my granddaughter, whose taste runs to *The Sound of Music*, and on particular, mostly nonmusical occasions, as when, one time, it helped to play simple duets with a very young patient new to my psychiatric office who was musical, and otherwise reluctant to engage.

In the spring of 2003, I drove to New York for the launch of my new book and a weekend of theatre. With a couple of hours between *Life x 3* and *Take Me Out*, I found myself on West Fifty-seventh Street, across the street from Carnegie Hall and, lo, the windows and doors of Steinway & Sons.

Somewhat automatically, almost as though hypnotized, I walked inside. A stream of amorphous, familiar, uncomfortable feelings that, mercifully, I had not felt in decades began to channel through. I felt like an impostor while, at the same time, I felt myself to be in a place I had abandoned where, really, I belonged. Awkwardly, I apologized to the approaching salesperson that I had no wish to buy a piano. In the kindest way, she invited me to browse through the rooms of instruments and left me to them.

Tentatively and then less so, I tried piano after piano. I found a couple that seemed clearly more comfortable and responsive than the others and whose tone I found pleasing— not overly brilliant, and more bell-like than wooden in the highest registers. I found one piano I liked very well. Price tag of $92,000. *I'd have to make a commitment to play and be willing to sacrifice other options to justify such a purchase.* With some sadness, with some resignation, and with some relief, I left. *Perhaps, in another lifetime . . .*

Three

Life-Giving Times

Graceful conches from tiny to good-sized sit on one sill, moon shells on another, of the windows in the foyer of my home. Scallop shells and moon shells perch on the desk and bookcase in my bedroom. One special moon shell has made it to the windowsill in the kitchen. A composition of black-and-white photographs by Andreas Feininger—shells shown in enlargement, a display of natural intricate geometric structure—fills a wall space in my piano room.

A feature of those life-giving days I spent each summer with my aunt and uncle in Harwichport, Cape Cod, was wading the shallow waters at low tide, searching for conch shells. I had a knack for finding them, some sort of built-in dowsing sense. I remember the excitement of reaching down into the sand and pulling up a heavy shell—sometimes heavy with the snail I could see pulling back and "spitting" sea water, other times heavy with grit and sand. The empty ones were certainly the prize. Conch snails were good for tickling, but once they closed up tight, the shell was not for keeping. Before I developed a conscience, I held on to one beauty for a couple of days, and the stink was pretty terrible. After that, live ones went back to the sea.

Sometimes Uncle Al took the boys and me fishing off the Herring River bridge. When I was nine, Fred was twelve and Neal was seven. Fred wasn't afraid to handle the creepy sea worms we used as bait—worms with a fringe of *legs*, worms that could *bite*. Uncle Al spent most of his time helping Neal and me, baiting our hooks and untangling our lines. One day we actually caught fish. We must have happened on a school of scup. One after the next small, flat, iridescent fish tugged on our lines and glinted in the sun as we reeled them in. Great excitement. There were enough for dinner, the sea had provided its bounty, and I felt like a pioneer.

Some weeks Uncle Al had to go back to Worcester to work. He'd take the car, and we could manage very well without one. Town was easy walking distance from our cottage. I wrote a postcard home every day, and each morning I could walk to the little post office to mail it. I remember being not much taller than counter height when I went to ask about any mail for me—and watched the postal lady remove the elastic band from a little packet of envelopes addressed to the houses on our street and flip through them one by one until she came to an envelope for *me*. I don't remember what the letters said, but the ritual of sending and receiving mail was a good-feeling connection to home.

We didn't need a car, either, to go to Snow Inn for dinner. We'd take a flashlight for safety after dark. I remember one moonless night: my aunt Bess leading the way with the flashlight, Fred at her side carrying his fishing rod, Neal and I following—Neal lugging a portable radio tuned to the Red Sox. A car approached, slowed, and stopped. The driver stuck his head out of the window and began to gesture and to laugh: "I thought you-all were a car with one headlight. It looked like the fishing pole was an antenna, and I heard the radio playing the ball game!"

Another sort of adventure was left to "the girls," the times when Auntie Bess and I would go "antiquing"—to Kathryn Sperry's shop, with its ruby glass shining through the windows, and the many shops on King's Highway. My favorite, though, was Windsong Antiques on Bank Street. The treasures there were housed in a building converted from a beautiful old barn. The proprietress was lovely and had the exotic name of Cassandra Bayliss. Over the years, Auntie Bess bought many pieces of china, some of which now are mine. In daily use, these plates, cups, and saucers bring the added pleasure of memories of those sweet days.

A couple of years ago, in November, I traveled to Hilton Head, invited by the South Carolina Academy of Family Physicians to speak about the role of testosterone in women's health. I found, happily, that the hotel where I was to stay faced directly at the ocean and featured a very long stretch of beach. My room was several floors up but oceanfront, with sliding glass doors leading out to a balcony. Having left the bare trees and early-winter weather of New England, I was delighted at the prospect of a walk in the sun by the sea. Unpacking could wait, and very soon I was barefoot on the white sand, enjoying the expanse of beach exposed at what happened just then to be low tide.

The shoreline featured an endless necklace of various types of snail shells, including moon shells in abundance. I had never seen so many of these magnificent dove-grey, satisfyingly round, whorled creations of nature. I picked up one after the next and, long since a purist in such matters, inspected each carefully for the presence of the snail. I collected a half dozen snail-less shells, about all I could carry, before returning to my hotel room, where I lined them up for a touch of home decoration on top of the dresser.

That night, I was partially wakened, a couple of times, by soft clicking sounds I half-consciously thought to be made by the clock. Waked fully by the early-morning sun, I noticed with some puzzlement that the dresser top was entirely bare. Could I believe my eyes? The moon shells were lined up along the bottom edge of the sliding glass doors. Hermit crabs, venturing out house-on-back in the night had, as a consequence of some mysterious natural tropism, crept out, dropped off the dresser, survived the fall, and made their way as near to the sea as they could manage. I couldn't wait to return them safely to the ocean.

This story has now become a *tell again, Gammy, about the moon shells* narrative requested by my granddaughter, who lives full-time on Cape Cod, and with whom I have the great pleasure of spending days by the shore. Alexandra and I collect shells, rescue starfish on South Beach from desiccation at low tide, and, most recently, enjoy cruising together on the small boat I bought for myself on the occasion of my sixty-fifth birthday. When I thought about naming this vessel, a name soon came to mind. I have named her *Windsong*.

Four

About God

"*F*ollow that will and that way which experience confirms to be your own," Carl Jung said. The truth of my experience is all I can manage, belief-wise. Still, from time to time, the truth of my experience has edged into a sense of something more.

Worcester, Massachusetts, 1943. I was four, that little Jewish girl in the huge extended family one generation from orthodoxy. My mother proudly told and retold the story of how *her* father had been so ecumenical and so kind as to establish the ritual of Christmas stockings for his eight American-born children, a ritual that carried down as my one taste of being like all the other kids in the neighborhood.

The rest of the year, I envied my friend Kathryn Rita Reilley, whose family went to mass (whatever that was) at Our Lady of Somethingsomething, and whose brother Bernie was becoming a priest. The mysteries of Ash Wednesday, when she and all the other kids had dirt put on their foreheads; cat-a-kissm classes taught by black-draped nuns with white-framed faces; and First Holy Communion—white dresses and white stockings and *white veils*—ah, none of these for me.

In first grade at Upsala Street School, I knew I must not cross myself or bow my head solemnly like Bernie Mattimore when we sang the name of Jesus in "Away in a Manger." My father cautioned me, with some measure of pride, that Jews must never bow to anyone except God—the God of the Jews, that is, *of whom we are the chosen people*. I did not understand what was so wonderful about being chosen.

But then there was Santa Claus. Incredibly, I was allowed Santa Claus. Christmas. The magic of colored lights framing eaves and doorways, draped over shrubs glowing in the blackness of the night, shining and twinkling through windows of the houses of Worcester's seven hills.

We couldn't have a tree. *Absolutely not, we're Jewish.* I never thought to question why it was that we *could* have a Christmas corner. And a corner it was, since no stocking could be hung by the chimney with care—we didn't have a fireplace. Our third-floor apartment in the three-decker didn't have central heat, for that matter. The kitchen stove ran on oil and was rigged to heat the room; the living room had an oil stove with a black enamel basin encrusted with residue from evaporated water sitting on the top of it. We closed off another room in the winter, because it just couldn't be heated. In a corner of the living room safely away from the stove, we made the Christmas corner. That is, Santa Claus made it.

On Christmas Eve, I left chocolate refrigerator cookies and a glass of milk with one of my knee socks next to it on the kitchen table and went to bed. In the morning, the milk had been drunk, the cookies were gone, and in the corner of the living room magic had happened. The floor was carpeted with layers of Christmas wrapping paper, upon which were piled a whole lot of presents, also Christmas-wrapped. My stocking was unrecognizable, stretched huge and lumpy with tangerines, walnuts, candy canes, and Hershey's Kisses. Best of all, everything dripped with tinsel, silver shining everywhere, almost as good as a tree. And every year, Santa dropped one present on his way out through the kitchen, in an awful rush, having so many children to take care of.

So to Christmas Eve 1943, when I am four years old. It is Friday night, *Shabbas*—the Sabbath—at my grandmother's house, in the kitchen with the green enamel Glenwood stove, the waxed linoleum, the maple table and chairs, the mahogany clock on the mantel that chimes and is wound with a key, and the radio with the war news. My mother, aunt, and grandmother have on cardigans over their patterned housedresses, and ankle socks with their laced up, black-for-winter, Cuban-heeled shoes. My father is, as he was required to do most Fridays, working late. After supper, when it's time for my mother and me to walk back up the hill to our home, Auntie Rosie looks into my face and says, "Sussaleh, you must be old enough

About God

now to know that there really isn't any Santa Claus." My chest feels cold. The night goes dead.

I don't remember much of the trek home, but when we are nearly there, *ohmygoodness . . . there . . . he . . . is*. Big and red and a shiny black belt and a bushy white beard and a hat and a sack. "Ho, ho, ho, little girl. You'd better get home and get to bed before I get there." I remember my mother dialing the telephone and putting me on with Auntie Rosie. "There is, too, Santa Claus. I just saw him."

Sometimes I wonder if this really happened, just as I wonder whether, once when I was snorkeling in the Caribbean, I really saw the sea horse holding by its tail to sea grasses. Evanescent moments of awe catch me unaware and are too much to hold—the truth of my experience, a wished-for challenge to agnosticism, but about what I can manage, belief-wise.

When I look back, I realize that God was a member of Bobba's household to whom I had not personally been introduced. Bobba mentioned him sometimes in Yiddish—*liebe Gott*, she would say, and I understood that that meant "dear God." From the earliest, I learned to understand Yiddish because that was what the grown-ups spoke when they didn't want me to know what they were saying. I kept to myself the truth that I did actually understand much more than the simple Yiddish phrases addressed to me.

These were, for the most part, blessings and curses. If I sneezed: *tsugezunt tsu lebn lang yore* (to health that you should live many years); if I burped: *grrepps heroise, gezunt hereine* (burp come out, health go in); and if I spilled some milk or dropped a piece of food on the floor, my mother would curse: *vayr fahgint dere nisht zoll alaine nisht hobben* (whoever may not wish you to have this morsel should himself be without). I still understand Yiddish, but if I try to speak, with the exception of the blessings and the curses, I cannot find the words. One crystal-cold day at Canon Mountain, when I was in my early thirties, I put on a pair of skis for the first (and last) time and, during the beginners' lesson, was astonished at the flow of Yiddish expletives and curses I heard coming from my mouth. It was as though I had become Bobba on skis—truly a wild idea, and the most memorable aspect of my day on the slopes.

During the years of my growing up, Bobba herself actually seldom left the house. On warm days, she might sit on the screened-in front porch and read the Yiddish newspaper or work on her crocheting. With a small, blunt crochet hook and what looked like a spool of twine she created lacy edging on linen bureau scarves, and made spider webs of doilies, antimacassars, and delicate tea aprons for her daughters and granddaughters. By the time I married, at twenty, doilies had had their day, but I have never been able to part with the dowry of crocheted items that Bobba made for me, still bearing the pink ribbons tied on by my mother to distinguish them from her own collection. As a loving symbol of her heritage, my daughter has one doily in a place of honor in her home.

When I think about how seldom Bobba ventured from the house, I remember that she went to shul (synagogue) only on Yom Kippur. Religiously, though, she prayed every day. Several times each day, in fact, she took down her worn prayer book from the kitchen mantelpiece, where it lay next to the clock, sat at the kitchen table, and prayed. I can still hear her murmur the Hebrew, see her lick her finger to turn a page, then close the book, kiss it, and return it to the mantel.

Each year, for many years, on Yom Kippur Bobba and I covered our heads with kerchiefs that she called *shalkes* and walked up the hill to the little shul, where we sat upstairs with the women. Downstairs the men, who wore black-and-white silk prayer shawls sometimes tented over their heads, stood and bobbed and rocked, murmured and chanted, notably not in unison. It was a noisily chaotic scene. Every once in a while, a man would call upstairs, not unkindly, to shush the women who might be chatting rather than praying, and to stage-whisper the page number in the prayer book they were supposed to be reading.

The shul was crowded with people who had not eaten and whose breath was not pleasant, and I was glad when we went out on the front steps for some fresh air. After a while, my mother or aunt would come to get me, but Bobba would stay until late in the day, when someone went to walk her home. Then, no matter that it was twilight, she refused to eat or drink until the streetlights went on—her sign that it was, officially, sunset. As Bobba aged, I wanted to call the power company on Yom Kippur to beg an earlier lighting of the streetlamps.

Such was the Jewish life of my family. As far as I knew, nobody but Bobba went to shul, and nobody else prayed. When I think about it, I know that my cousins Son and Mally must have been bar mitzvahed, but that was before my time. When I was nine or ten, my parents scraped together the money to send me to Sunday school at Temple Emanuel on the west side, the better part of the city—across town from the blue-collar, mostly Catholic part of the east-side neighborhood where we lived. I didn't know one person in religious school class and was lonely and miserable. Sometimes the boys chased around wildly, lobbing bagels at one another, and when I complained about this to my parents, to my relief, they let me quit.

Within a year or so, in 1949, the postwar housing shortage taught me the meaning of eviction. Our landlord needed our apartment for some member of his family back from the service, and my parents had a hard time finding another place for us to live. The upshot was that we moved three times and I attended four different schools in four years before my parents managed to buy a two-family house where we settled down a couple of blocks from Temple Emanuel. The former bagel-lobbing boys were now my classmates in ninth grade at Chandler Junior High, and Temple Emanuel became, for me at least, a center for Jewish social activity more than for spiritual experience.

Although I was, literally, a new kid on the block, adolescence was new territory for everybody, and I found myself at no particular disadvantage. I was present from the first for the Saturday night ballroom-dancing classes and, on the whole, enjoyed them, dressed up like the other girls in swirly skirts with crinoline petticoats cinched in at the waist by wide elastic belts, and layered, from the skin out, with a garter belt holding up nylon stockings with seams up the back, or a panty girdle holding in a barely discernible belly. Periodically I wore another kind of belt, with W-shaped attachers for the gauze extensions of sanitary napkins. All of this trussing up, while not exactly comfortable, felt excitingly grown-up, as did the lipstick and the medium-high-heeled pumps I was allowed to wear.

At Temple Emanuel, too, I attended enough Sabbath services with Bar Mitzvah ceremonies and enough annual High Holiday services to become familiar with Hebrew prayers and choral music. I found some of the music beautiful and some of the prayers rhythmically appealing, but I felt nothing else I could have identified as spiritual.

What did stir me was the charisma and sensuality of the young rabbi whose first congregation after ordination, in 1953, was Temple Emanuel in Worcester, where he stayed for six years. Only fourteen years older than the ninth-graders who were my peers, Rabbi Alexander Schindler seemed always to be surrounded by clamoring teenage kids who called him "Alex." I longed to as well, but I never dared approach him at all.

I wish I had.

At services, I had an unfamiliar feeling in my heart and belly when I listened to him chant the Kaddish. I remember him standing in his black robe, face uplifted and eyes closed, rocking back and forth on his heels and chanting the Hebrew words as though he could taste them. I suppose that's what "savoring words" must mean.

I am not a daily reader of the *New York Times*, and rarely scan its obituaries. Chance had it that, five years ago, while visiting my sweetheart in upstate New York, I picked up the paper at breakfast on a Thursday morning and read:

RABBI ALEXANDER SCHINDLER
1925–2000

Rabbi Alexander Schindler, leader of the Reform movement of American Judaism for a quarter of a century, died at his Westport, Connecticut, home November 15, 2000, shortly after marking his 75th birthday . . .

Sadness welled up, and regret for opportunities missed began to wash in. The adolescent girl I was fifty years past wouldn't have conceived the question, but now I wanted to know what Rabbi Schindler might say about God. Subsequently I searched and managed to find a collection of essays written by others in Schindler's honor. Published while he lived, in 1995, each essay was introduced by an excerpt of a speech or a sermon of Schindler's. In one of these I found his words:

> When our children feel the budding of compassion, the swelling of love, the sorrow of repentance, it is then that we must say to them: "Ah, now you are standing in the presence of God."

I found another passage, in the postscript to the essays, that told me more about Rabbi Schindler's personal faith:

> Words like despair and gloom, hopelessness and doom are not part of my life's vocabulary. And what if reason dictates otherwise? Then reason must be transcended, for when the phi-

losopher postulates, "I think, therefore I am," the Jew within
me emphatically replies, "I believe, therefore I live."

I'm afraid that I was raised on a formula with too many parts desperation and too few parts belief to nourish the faith of the Jew within me. When my mother's Polish friend Bette made a novena asking for divine intervention in my college application process, the full scholarship I was granted to Wellesley was to me more evidence of Bette's love than of God's. Rabbi Schindler might well have told me that they were one and the same.

At Wellesley, the two required courses were Freshman English and, of all things, Biblical History. Bible stories, that is, Old Testament Bible Stories—about Joseph and his Coat of Many Colors or Ruth in the Barley Fields—had been among my childhood books, but I had never read the Bible. The required textbook for class was the Revised Standard Version, which, of course, included the New Testament. Jesus. Not much had changed for me since first-grade Christmas carols. I wasn't sure that a Jew was allowed to have a Bible like that. The Old Testament took up the first 997 pages, all small print, and when I found that Matthew, Mark, Luke, and John appeared to be near the end of the book, I was relieved, because I figured that at least we wouldn't get to them for a while.

But soon I had a different problem. I discovered that the Old Testament, with its god who demanded singular commitment and with all its wars and punishments, frightened me. Earnest discussions in dorm late-night talks with the junior girls who were majoring in Biblical History brought forth the idea of "the leap of faith" required to believed in God. I just couldn't get that far off the ground. Caught between my lack of faith and a coexisting fear that this retributive god might read my thoughts, I was tormented by the blasphemous idea that the god of the Jews seemed pretty insecure—having to order us not to worship any other gods and not trusting that we could just love him. My ambivalence expresses itself today in the uncertainty I have about capitalizing the "g" in *god*—a problem not resolvable by Strunk and White.

In the spring of sophomore year at Wellesley, someone stuck a flower and a little slip of paper saying *God Is Love* into the name-tag holders on the doors of our dorm rooms. A tiny footnote referenced the Gospel of John for what I learned was Christianity's central metaphor. I hadn't yet found anything like "God Is Love" in the Old Testament, and I wasn't then equipped with Rabbi Schindler's affirmation that, for Jews too, love means the presence of God.

A couple of decades after I graduated from college, hoping to connect with some spiritual experience in the religion of my roots, I joined a class studying the Jewish mystical tradition of Kabala. This was not the New Age version. We met in an old synagogue near Central Square in Cambridge and were taught by a serious young rabbi imported from Israel. Alexander Schindler he was not. He drew a lot of circles on a paper and spoke in a didactic and solemn manner about each of us being a spark split off from the Divine and longing to return to the Source. His dry discourse did not inspire feeling.

What did inspire thought was his description of the different levels of giving and receiving. I remember the rabbi saying that the "lowest" level was:

Receiving for the sake of receiving.

A more worthy combination was:

Giving for the sake of receiving.

Next in the hierarchy was:

Giving for the sake of giving.

So far so good. Okay, I can and *do* do that. But when he described the only remaining and most exalted permutation, I knew I was done for:

Receiving for the sake of giving.

I do not even aspire to that degree of generosity. I know that I am lacking in grace, but if I don't want something, I don't want it.

Then the rabbi told us that we could break all the rules of Kabala for nearly the whole of our lifetime, but if we kept to them strictly for the last twelve months of our life, we would be home free, so to speak. He meant it. I wondered if perhaps this was some angle on divine forgiveness and absolution, but decided that more likely the apparent loophole was a wry manipulation. After all, we cannot predict with absolute certainty when we will die. If the rabbi's intention was to convey to us that it was never too late to begin to follow the laws of Kabala and to inspire us to try, I'm afraid he failed with me. I had had enough of this, and I dropped the class.

The matter of belief and of prayer came up for serious consideration nine years ago, when I was fifty-six, and several months after my father died. Although he had been raised in an Orthodox Jewish home, my dad was, in his life, not so much adherently religious as creative in his rituals. Particularly in his later years (I don't remember him doing so while I lived at home), he meditated, communed, and prayed in his own way.

My dad once told me that, in his dreams, he could fly. While dreaming, he would see and feel himself walking forward and simply taking off into the air, as naturally as breathing. I understand very well what he meant, because I have such dreams. My dreams of flying have been so vivid that in waking life I occasionally feel as though I should be able to propel myself easily into the air.

Since I could not propel myself easily into prayer, while he lived I relied on my dad to take care of that for me. The spring after he died, in 1996, I began to feel uneasy about my neglect in the prayer department. So I did what I customarily do—read books and consult experts. My memory of Rabbi Schindler was at that time buried along with the other unmet longings of my childhood. Had I thought of it, I would have tried to contact him—a missed opportunity about which today I have regret. The best I could manage at the time was to read

Heschel, which wasn't of much use, and to speak with a couple of local rabbis, to no greater avail.

Help did finally come during an afternoon talk with a friend I had met in a serendipitous way—via a circuitous networking effort that could be said to have been influenced by a divine hand. Myrna, who is experienced in the book world, is as much retired as her passion for the work and the importuning of authors will permit. I met her in 1994 when, having spent three years on the project, I was stuck in my efforts to find a way to broadcast the information I had discovered about testosterone deficiency and supplementation for women. When I pestered writers at *Boston Magazine* for referral to an effective public relations person, what do you know? They sent me to one—who responded to my call with an invitation to meet for a drink at the Parker House, listened to my story, looked at my work, and suggested that I call Myrna ("You'll love each other"). Myrna showed up at our first meeting with a list of prospective agents for my prospective book, which was sold to a major publisher four months later. Considering what it takes to get a book published, a case could be made for a miracle here.

The following year, after my dad died and during the time of my unease about prayer, Myrna and I got together for one of our country drives and rambling talks. When I brought up the matter of prayer, she said, "Well, we can start with what we know, and we do know that telepathy occurs. Prayer is a way of communicating with the world telepathically."

I know that some psychiatrists would smack a label of

"magical thinking" on the idea of a telepathic network that operates on a power grid we can't learn about in physics. I am not one of them. Leap of faith? I can't do it. Telepathy? Piece of cake. Go figure. I suppose it's that Jungian thing—"believe only the truth of your experience." Person-to-person communication without contact has always been as real to me as the air I breathe. Apparently, when it's a person-to-person(s) matter, transcending reality to the extent of a nonphysical power grid is within my scope. Relating to people present or absent is at the core of my life. But god? Well, Bobba could do it, but I can't speak directly to *liebe Gott*. It has been a gift that, ever since Myrna framed the matter of prayer as telepathic communication with the universe, I have been able to pray—to speak from my heart to the good in humanity, to whom I can send strength, inspiration, light, thoughts, blessings, and from whom sometimes I can ask help. I have found that at critical occasions when I could otherwise do nothing, as when I received news of the extended labor and risk at the birth of my grandchild, sending every telepathic message possible out to the universe comforted me. Then, when the baby was safely born, what do you know, I thanked God.

It seems that I can more readily thank God than expect God to listen to anything else I might say. Maybe God is the recipient of some really lousy unresolved transference. By their own assertions, my parents didn't know what to make of me. My lack of faith could be simply that I can't imagine a dependable source of love that could understand my heart and mind.

Not having had dependably empathic parents is rather a common experience, though, and not everybody who gets short shrift in parenting ends up an atheist or an agnostic. When I ran this by my good friend Allen, he offered that "those people who have the will to take care of themselves don't turn to God." There's something to that, but it's not pat. Several of my close friends, men and women who clearly do have the will to take care of themselves, still do commune with God (one of them communes with goddesses), yet few had notably empathic parents. Then, too, there are those who don't have the will to take care of themselves and who don't turn to God, but to drugs, alcohol, food, sex . . .

I think back to Jung's dictum. "Believe only the truth of your experience" gave him plenty of latitude, for sure. Jung wrote of having visions, of tinkering with alchemy, and of states of consciousness and realms of experience unfamiliar to most of us. In the documentary film *A Matter of Heart,* Jung's student Dr. Maria Luisa von Franz recounted this delightful anecdote (transcribed exactly as spoken):

> One of the last times he [Jung] went to the tower [his country home] he hadn't been there for a long time, and the first days, the covers of the pans liked to jump off and fall on the floor at the wrong moments and . . . you know how objects can absolutely misbehave. So he put himself out in the middle of the kitchen and said: "Now, ladies and gentlemen, pots and pans, spoons—I know I have neglected you for a long time, and you are angry with me. But I beg your pardon, and I ask you now to cooperate again." And from then on, there were no more accidents. He had great fun with that.
>
> If you notice, it's highly symbolic the days you can't open

a door, you can't get at something, some object hides from you—generally when you are not in yourself—and in an impatient mood or so on. Then everything plays you tricks. It's naturally your own unconscious mixed up with it, but it [your unconscious] communicates with matter.

I don't speak to my cutlery, but I am drawn to some modalities of healing that transcend the limits of what we can prove—methods such as Reiki, "hands-on" healing. While I am not, at heart, a skeptic, the truth is that I approached my first experience of Reiki with some skepticism, focused not so much on the method as on the particular practitioner.

At the time, I was suffering from pain caused by an inflammation in my jaw joint. The mechanics of the problem had resulted in a period of time when I could neither open my mouth freely nor close my mouth fully. I was really miserable. It hurt even to speak. I think I did some of my best psychiatric work during that time, since the pain resulted in my being extraordinarily selective in what I chose to say, and my unfamiliar passivity pushed my patients to do more of their own work than was for them customary.

Having consulted Boston's medical and dental experts, I chose the conservative course of learning to relax my jaw and giving my body time to heal. It hurt to chew, so I lost some weight. That was okay. Although I had resigned myself to living with it, the pain was wearing. Finally, figuring I had nothing to lose, I took up the many-times-repeated offer of an eccentric member of my social bridge group and presented myself to him for a session of Reiki.

I had never felt comfortable with Don. He had been married, had made his fortune young, had divorced, and now seemed to be a vigilantly independent person. Don was a loner committed to being true to himself, no matter the impact on others. In circumscribed ways, he was very generous. He delivered meals to the elderly; he did Reiki at no charge. But in the realm of less boundaried social exchange, he was prepared to put his needs first, and he counted on others to watch out for themselves. There was integrity in this, but it didn't generate trust. Don seemed an unlikely person to be a healer.

At the first session, I found the laying on of hands to be at best restful and at worst boring. The procedure required only that I lie fully clothed on a massage table while Don placed his hands on each of six or so prescribed (and certainly not proscribed) places on my body. He quietly kept contact in each position for, I guessed, ten minutes or so—about an hour in all. I felt nothing.

After the second session, the pain in my jaw . . . simply . . . disappeared . . .

So did Don, from time to time, as he followed his avocation as a semiprofessional athlete. A couple of years later, when my back acted up, I tracked down another Reiki practitioner—one more personable, empathic, and warm. She was a lovely person. But she didn't turn out quite to have Don's power, whatever that might have been.

My psychiatric work with patients is, for the most part, traditional. Occasionally I find that some creative modality helps stimulate access to the heart of a matter otherwise blocked. I have used Carol B. Anthony's interpretation of the *I Ching* as a facilitator. Her way in to the universal wisdom of this ancient text dependably brings helpful perspective to any circumstance. Some time ago I studied with Richard Allen, a teacher of a Cherokee shamanic practice of guided meditation. He was experienced in a method of active imagination used to invoke an animal or a person, who would come to mind "to provide wisdom for the next step in one's growing."

For all of our sessions but the last, Richard and I met at his teaching space. We had our final meeting at my office, which occupies most of the ground floor of the large Victorian house that has been my home for the past thirty-seven years. Immediately on entering the consulting room, Richard began to stare at the wall behind my chair.

"What's behind there?"

"The back staircase leading up to the second floor."

"Can we take a look to see what's there?"

We found Jasper, the beloved fourteen-year-old Cairn terrier who'd become a member of our household when he was a puppy and my daughter, Jennifer, was twelve. He was lying dead on the bottom step.

My memory of the uncanny discovery is a blur of shock, sadness, and gratitude. Jasper had been showing his age for some time, but he had been pretty frisky just the night before, running around the house, barking happily, and begging treats from my bridge group. I felt sad for my loss, but even sadder for Jennifer's. Jasper had been her dog since he was a puppy, and she loved him as much as a girl can love a dog. It might be true that she loved him as much as a girl can love, period. Jennifer's husband, Tom, had once semiseriously observed that Jasper just might be on the receiving end of more affection than he.

As for the gratitude I felt: with the suddenness of Jasper's death, I could think that he might not have suffered much; no debilitating illness had required any anguishing decision making at the end; and, certainly, Richard's sensitivity to *who-knows-what* provided the blessing of his company in this sad event.

While I contacted Jenni at her summer workplace and she reached Tom at his, Richard began to chant the Tibetan prayers for the dead. When the two of them arrived, Richard was still chanting. The prayer ritual continued while Tom dug a grave and Jenni and I wrapped Jasper in a sheet. All of us buried him.

Jenni said the only words I remember: *"Dear God, please take care of Jasper."*

Ahhhhhhh. Jasper's great gift to me. I learned that the daughter I had raised could speak to God.

Five

Alone, Together, Alone

*I*n 1956 *it's time for me to do something about college. Nei-*
ther of my parents had had the opportunity. Nobody in my extended family did either, except for my cousin Noah, who had
gone to Clark on the G.I. Bill. We have no money for tuition,
so I figure I'll apply to Clark, hope for a scholarship, live at
home, and commute by bus. I think I should have a good
chance: my school report cards note that I have earned "all
A's" since kindergarten, except for a B in effort, once. (My
father likes to say, *What do they mean—she got all A's without
trying?*) Although I'm not a National Merit scholar, I have
earned a Certificate of Merit (*given to the top one-tenth of one*

percent of the graduating high school seniors in the U.S., my mother quotes repeatedly from the accompanying letter until she has it memorized, and so do I). The guidance counselor urges me to apply to at least one additional college. I am thinking a lot about the fact that next year will be Julie's last at Clark, and we want to be able to continue to spend time together. Finally I decide to apply to Wellesley, which is only about thirty miles away.

In May 1957, the acceptance letters arrive. Tuition at Clark is six hundred dollars, and they've granted me a partial scholarship. Tuition, room, and board at Wellesley is fifteen hundred and fifty dollars, and Wellesley has offered a full scholarship— requiring only that I work on campus several hours per week. As unlikely a development as it is, it turns out that I can better afford to go to Wellesley. I don't really know what to expect, but I am pretty excited. So is my family. Bobba, in particular, is very happy that I am going to go to "Velsel."

Wellesley gives me a choice of rooms, single or double. I am sure that I need privacy. I know I will be risking loneliness, but I'm used to that. What concerns me more is the possibility that having a roommate might require stressful accommodation. I choose a single. In truth, this consideration could be said to be the pattern from which my life continues to be cut to this day.

My room at the end of a corridor in Davis Hall turns out to be the last in a series of freshman singles. I bless the fates that decreed the room next to mine be assigned to someone who, virtually as soon as we meet, presses on me her copy of *The Catcher in the Rye* to read and discuss, the beginning of a friendship that will know no end. It comes to pass that Linda and I talk about everything—mundane to existential. She and I have had quite different upbringings, but at heart we are very much in sync. I am impressed with some of her attributes of sophistication—she smokes Marlboros, she drinks Scotch (on dates, and not much, but still . . .), her clothes come from Bergdorf's, her family has a maid and a chauffeur at their Long Island home and a penthouse apartment on Fifth Avenue, she has attended a boarding school in France, at Chamonix—but I am all the more impressed that the goal of her life is to help the disadvantaged.

Linda worked the previous summer as a counselor at a camp for crippled kids. During our freshman year at Wellesley, she volunteers to paint slum apartments in Roxbury with the students from Phillips Brooks House at Harvard, and when Fidel Castro comes to Cambridge she joins the crowd at the rally in Harvard Square. She aims, ultimately, to become a social worker.

I am impressed also that every day and Sunday, Linda reads the *New York Times*—something of a different rag from the *Worcester Telegram and Gazette* and the *Jewish Civic Leader*. I try to read the *Times* but find the effort daunting—like trying to understand a book I've begun in the middle.

For her part, Linda is impressed that I am not freaked out by my scholarship work, the more so as the particular task has been of my own choosing. (Twice each week I'm responsible for cleaning the cages and refilling the water bottles of rats that are kept in the dark for an experiment by a biology professor.) Other details of Linda's initial experience of me (of which

I have no idea at the time): she finds me exotic and, actually, "terrifying." This latter is a function of my eschewing the wearing of a girdle (!) and my offhand comment that Linda's girdle "makes her into a sausage." I don't realize that I am on sensitive ground; her mother has warned her about the dangers of going on dates without such armor. I never guess that Linda glances at my untethered body with alarm and envy when, on weekends, I dress for a date with Julie.

An extensive and comfortable arena does exist for Linda and me. We share a fascination with the life of the mind and the life of the emotions. Late into the night, many nights, we talk, and talk, and talk. Having never before known what it is to be seen and understood clearly and enjoyed for being myself, I begin really to come to know myself and feel fully alive for the first time in my life.

My new and wonderful friendship does begin to create some problems, though. Within a few months, Julie begins to be jealous of the enthusiasm I express when I talk about Linda. I'm a little puzzled, since there is no romantic element to the friendship. Julie's unhappiness creates disquietude for me. I begin to wonder if maybe something really might be missing between him and me. I've been wearing his pearl-and-gold Phi Alpha fraternity pin for a couple of years, which means that we've been "going steady." Next year he'll be going halfway across the country to begin medical school at the University of Cincinnati. With the prospect of being apart for most of the next four academic years, I am actually relieved when we come to the decision that, when Julie leaves for medical school, we will give ourselves the freedom to date other people.

Sophomore year begins as a real adventure. No single for me this time: Linda and I are rooming together. We won a choice number in the room lottery and are enjoying a two-room suite in Claflin Hall, a dormitory on the quadrangle at Tower Court. It's not really all that grand, but we've put both our beds in one small room, both our desks in the other, and it's almost like an apartment. Small windows crank open to look out over Lake Waban, particularly beautiful as it reflects the autumn foliage.

Early that fall my cousin Fred, who is a student at the Massachusetts College of Pharmacy, introduces me to the older brother of a girl he is dating. Jordy and I enjoy meeting and start to date, but before long the pressure begins. Saturday night after Saturday night I return to the dorm from an evening out with Jordy to find a collage of notes with my name on them tacked to the "bell board," the telephone message board—all of them from Julie. He is clearly frantic that I am out with someone else.

The rest of this story is painful to tell. In February, in desperation, Julie actually petitions my mother to intercede on his behalf. Linda remembers more vividly than I my mother's coming to the dorm to persuade me to commit myself exclusively to Julie. I am nauseous when I think of her interference. It can be said that when he and I began to connect, my mother passed the baton for my welfare to Julie. When I dared to risk letting go of him, the two of them came forward together. And I caved. I wasn't ready for marriage to *anybody*, and neither was he. In the words of my future mentor, Dr. Elvin Semrad:

The more mature a relationship, the more able the two people are to give up their dependency and learn how to live alone together.

At that time, Julie and I still had a lot to learn about how to live independently.

Semrad put it another way:

You can only be close when you're separate.

By the time I managed to develop myself sufficiently separate both from my parents and from Julie, I had been in the marriage for several years and had had a child. Although my husband and I earnestly tried to be loving and helpful to each other, it wasn't in the cards for him and me to be close in an alive way. I could not thrive in this union.

Although ultimately the marriage failed, I do not hold regrets. It helped me grow away from the influence of my mother and come more into my own. It gave me the great gift of my daughter and, eventually, of my granddaughter. I cherish many of the early memories of the connection to my childhood sweetheart, and I accept that, like all things that come to pass in a life lived to the best of one's abilities, it could not have been otherwise.

Six

Scientific
Foundations

*T*wo *years before I quit the piano, I took my first stand to* be allowed to let go of something. It happened like this: Worcester public school had three "tracks": vocational, general or commercial, and prep for college. The college-prep track required French in seventh grade and added Latin in eighth. I loved French, but Latin . . . oh, I detested it. One year's basic vocabulary was enough for me to learn what I found interesting about the roots of other languages, but declensions and grammar were tedious, and translating passages about Caesar's military campaigns felt useless and boring. I begged to be allowed to drop Latin and to take in its place

Physiology and Health, an elective that was offered to the "general" students. Wonder of wonders . . . I got my wish.

Studying for that course, learning how our bodies work, reading about the circulation of the blood through the heart and to the lungs, about lymph, about blood corpuscles, about the function of the spleen, about the ovaries and the uterus and the menstrual cycle, and the names of all the bones in the body, I had the odd experience that I was reconnecting with material that was already, somehow, familiar to me. My interest in all of this mirrored that of my dad, who had a notable zest for life in general and for knowledge of the natural world in particular.

Self-taught, my dad had accumulated a fund of miscellaneous, obscure, and mostly accurate information, which he passed on whenever an opportunity even obliquely presented itself. His material ranged from knowledge about the wasp that is essential to the life cycle of the fig (to this day, I look for a trace when I take a crunchy bite), to geological curiosities like isinglass, and to stories about an English uncle who invented a World War I gas-mask filter made out of prune pits and was supposedly knighted for this achievement. I can't bring myself to go to the reference library microfiche on that one.

My favorite times with my dad happened before I was five, in the years before he came to own the grocery store that swallowed him up. In those earlier years, he used to take me, paper bag with stale Jewish bread in hand, to Green Hill Park to feed the carp. I remember standing next to him on the mossy bank of the lake, our bread floating patiently on the water, and then . . . the excitement of watching huge fish with great open mouths swim slowly up to the surface, take in a whole soggy slice in one gulp, and then turn with a splash of tail to dive down deep into the lake again.

Leisure to play with me ended with the mixed blessing of my dad coming to own his own grocery store. This happened in some "special" way, the details of which were never fully explained to me. As a child, I heard that Manny Seagull (Siegel), the son of our elderly landlady, appreciated that my parents looked after his mother, who lived downstairs, and so Manny in some way helped my dad buy from him a property with an empty store. I used to think that the Seagulls had simply given the store to my father as a reward for my parents' kindness—sort of like the pot of gold that the good little child (depicted in my book of fables and morality tales) found when he moved the huge rock in the road. At the time, my parents didn't have money for a down payment on anything, and I imagine that Manny made an arrangement for my dad to buy the store without one.

What I remember of old Mrs. Seagull has to do with a particular lampshade of hers. I was, at the time, three years old. Many an afternoon, my mother joined Mrs. Seagull for tea in her kitchen, while I (*Sussaleh's so good, she's quiet as a mouse*) amused myself in the living room by stripping the tiny colored glass beads off the fringe of a most wonderful lampshade. A magical shimmer came from the fallen beads—red, blue, amber—on the dark carpet. One of those days when I was busily working away—some fringes remained yet to debead—I was discovered, alas, and the Seagull living room was off-limits after that.

My dad came to own his store in 1944, when the civilian impact of World War II included food rationing. I remember the small, round, sturdy, red and blue glossy cardboard tokens that my dad collected along with the cash for rationed purchases. Meat, in particular, was rationed—both to the customers and to the stores that sold it. Before he opened Robert's Market, my father's experience had been in selling produce and dairy. Having had no training as a butcher, he came up with an ingenious and exhausting arrangement with a purveyor (I think it was Chicago Dressed Beef Company) to work as an apprentice in exchange both for learning how to break down sides of beef and for the privilege of buying meat to sell. For a year, my dad got up each day at four in the morning to cut meat for the wholesale butcher, then returned to run his own market from eight A.M. until dark.

From that time on, the only place I spent any quality time with my dad was in his store. This wasn't a total loss. He radiated energy, and he loved to show me his skills at designing and drawing signs, at setting up food displays, and at engaging the customers. While he didn't sell snow to the Eskimos, my father's resourcefulness as a marketer could be imaginative. One particular episode became legend. Foundational facts: most of my dad's customers were neighborhood regulars, well known to him; Robert's Market, at the quiet corner of Vernon and Esther Streets, did not enjoy much drive-by, drop-in business; fish was not a popular food except on Fridays, when observant Catholics abstained from eating meat.

One Friday, as my dad told it, he had sold the last of his supply of fish to a familiar customer, who had cooked it and, deciding that the haddock didn't taste "right" to her, had brought back the cooked fish for a refund. Shortly, a car pulled up and a woman he hadn't seen before came into the store asking to buy some fresh fish. Having no more to sell, my dad came up with the idea to offer the woman his "special cooked haddock," which she purchased at some premium price. He considered himself lucky and clever—that is, until the following Friday, when that same car pulled up and that same woman came out, asking to buy some more of that "delicious special cooked haddock."

I wasn't on hand for the haddock incident, but I did spend a lot of time in the store after school, when my mother sometimes helped out at the cash register while my dad waited on customers at the meat counter. The back room of the store had the hamburg grinder, an electric vertical bone saw, a meat-cutting block worn crooked by generations of butchers wire-brush-scouring its surface, and a walk-in freezer.

Watching my dad cut meat became my first class in vertebrate anatomy. Standing back at a safe distance, and with great interest, I learned where tenderloin steaks, sirloin steaks, and rib roasts originate. I believe that it was the pleasure I experienced in my connection to my dad, together with the evident respect he had for life and the care and pride he took in his work, that overrode whatever disturbing connections I might otherwise have made between the animals in my books and the carcasses in the back room. In my calling to medicine, in truth, my dad was my first mentor.

Passion for natural science and for teaching are qualities that have drawn me to several of the most important men in my life. I come to meet the one next most significant, after my dad, in June 1958, after my sophomore year at Wellesley, when I find a summer job at the Worcester Foundation for Experimental Biology in Shrewsbury, Massachusetts—along with my hometown friend Irma, who goes to Simmons College. The Worcester Foundation, where Gregory Pincus and Hudson Hoagland have been developing the birth control pill, is a happening place these days. Other researchers are doing experiments with something called LSD. Sometime later that summer, in the interest of science and for something like twenty dollars, Irma volunteers to take it. She cannot exactly describe her experience, and I do not exactly understand it. She seems to enjoy it, however.

I am busy with my work as a lab assistant to Dr. Harris Rosenkrantz, who is studying the effects of vitamin E deficiency on the adrenal glands of rabbits. My first exposure to neuroendocrine research involves colorimetric assays to measure something that taps off my tongue: "five-hydroxy-tryptamine." This compound has another, smoother name: serotonin. Nobody has any idea that Prozac and other drugs to regulate serotonin will become aspirin for depression a couple of decades down the road. At nineteen, I have never even met a psychiatrist and have no idea that I will ever be one.

That summer, engaged to be married to Julie, I am living at home in Worcester—a long, many-transfers bus commute from the lab. It happens that Dr. Rosenkrantz lives, with his wife and two small sons, only a few streets away from my parents, and helpfully offers me a lift to work each morning. He drives a standard-transmission car and I, who got headaches taking driving lessons on a standard and finked out to learn on Julie's automatic, am impressed that he is a skillful driver. I notice that he both drives and shifts with his right hand, steadying the wheel with his right forearm, but I don't give this much of a thought. Some days I have to fend for myself getting home, because Dr. Rosenkrantz plays tennis at Clark University with some colleagues after work.

In our lab, there are two permanent lab assistants. One is very pregnant. The other is French-Canadian, Roland Le-something—"Rolie." Dr. Rosenkrantz sometimes joins in the lab work, deft with a pipette—always with his left hand in his left pants pocket. This gives him a sort of relaxed and casual look. All I make of it is that, like the driving, he is more ex-perienced and better at it than am I. Certainly I see how a research scientist who keeps hands on in the laboratory can know for himself what his technicians are doing.

Dr. Rosenkrantz is very clear about laboratory protocol and technique. He teaches and I learn about "safety solutions"— huge plastic bottles, called carboys, of dilute acid and base kept near the sink to neutralize spilled alkali or acid in the event of accident. That summer I also learn some other things. Al-though I am assured that a humane way to sacrifice rabbits— *they don't even know what hit them*—is to slam them on the head with a wrench, I find that I cannot, myself, do it. I learn that Taufik El Atar, the Egyptian scientist who works in the lab next to ours, is very attractive and appears to wear clear finger-nail polish on his manicured fingernails. And one day, as I am standing next to Dr. Rosenkrantz, I notice in the gap above the wrist cuff button of his long-sleeved shirt that the flesh of his left arm looks peculiar.

After that glimpse in the gap of the sleeve, I go over to Rolie's bench. "What's the matter with Dr. Rosenkrantz's arm?" Rolie doesn't look up from what he's doing. "Harris doesn't have a left arm. He doesn't have a left leg, either. New York City subway accident, when he was a kid."

My brain races to make sense of what I knew yet hadn't known. Dr. Rosenkrantz regularly smokes a pipe. I remember sitting across the desk from him, going over lab data while he, most naturally and so often, with his one hand, automatically filled the bowl inside the pouch, put the pipe into his mouth and held it at an angle with his back teeth clenched, tamped, and lit it. And it had never occurred to me that . . .

I think some more. While his gait is distinctive, Dr. Rosenkrantz doesn't actually limp. How does he play tennis? Later, once, I get to watch. With his one arm and hand, he holds the racket, bounces and hits the ball to serve, then moves around the court in doubles play, hitting well enough sometimes to win. All things considered, I think that his quite beautiful wife, Natalie, and their two little boys have a husband and father more whole than many. This extraordinary summer experience comes to an end. I am given a going-away party, complete with a hand-lettered certificate decorated in the corners with illustrations of rabbits and wrenches. I will never forget any of it.

Three years later, in June 1961, I have graduated college, Julie and I have married, and we are living in Cincinnati,

Ohio, while he completes his last year of medical school. We plan that when Julie graduates, we will move back east for him to begin training in pediatrics and for me, I hope, to begin medical school. For this year, I take a job as a laboratory assistant at an institute for medical research.

I am hired by Dr. P., whose plan it is that I learn tissue-culture technique from the departing lab technician. The assay is designed to measure the growth in test tubes of tissue obtained from kidneys transplanted from one dog to another. The first day, I follow along to learn the painstaking steps in the process. We begin by swabbing the laboratory floor with an iodine antiseptic and spraying the air with an ozone disinfectant. We finish up by measuring the density of color in our final sample tubes, an indicator of the amount of tissue present in each tube. That part is familiar; I did that for Dr. Rosenkrantz.

At the end of a long day's work, when we place tube after tube in the colorimeter, the needle on the indicator dial barely moves: .001, a virtually insignificant reading. Scratches on the tubes could account for it. Puzzled, I tell the lab technician who will soon be leaving this job to me, "There's nothing in these tubes." He says, "Uh, that's okay. We'll just cover them, leave them on top of the refrigerator, and we'll read them again tomorrow."

Sure enough, the next day we read the tubes again. This time, the readings are edging into significance. By the fourth day, we really have something to show for all this effort. And I think that we probably have other things growing in the tubes as well. Maybe even mushrooms. I have no doubt that after spending half a week on top of the laboratory refrigerator, these tubes are contaminated, and that the growing contaminants are, in fact, what we have been measuring. With this, I am now on my own.

Dr. P. never sets foot in the laboratory. He spends much of his time masked and suited up in green scrubs in an operating room, where he and an assistant do kidney-transplant surgery on dogs. The scuttlebutt is that Dr. P. is a frustrated would-be surgeon who didn't make it into medical school. Here he gets to operate on dogs, though. That's where the kidney tissue comes from that I am trying to culture and measure.

When I meet with him in his office to discuss my work, it appears that the many days' readings of tubes sitting on top of the refrigerator is news to him. I wonder: *Have research papers been written based on this data?* I feel sick when I think, *Dogs have been sacrificed to obtain this data.* I have no idea whether the results of the painstaking work I will be doing will be comingled with data based on contaminated assays. I decide, in any event, that I will record only one day's readings on any tissue culture assay that I run.

In a gesture of accommodation to my standards, Dr. P. gives me free rein with the requisition book. I am determined to try, at least, to run a proper lab. None of the procedures I am called upon to do requires the use of chemical acids or alkalis. Still, I learned from Dr. Rosenkrantz, whose presence and integrity I miss more than a little, that every laboratory must be equipped with safety solutions. I order carboys. I make safety solutions. I do tissue cultures. I run assays. The tubes continue to read .001. Zilch.

Several times each week my lab procedure requires the use of a candle filter—a hollow, unglazed porcelain cylinder that looks like a thick white candle but is open at one end. To use it, I attach the filter by means of a rubber cork to a heavy-walled, flat-bottomed flask hooked up to a strong vacuum pump. The solution to be filtered is pulled by vacuum through the porcelain, where any tiny particle will be trapped.

After use, both candle filters and fine-bored glass pipettes are cleaned by the laboratory person hired as "dishwasher," who stands them upright, open ends at the bottom, in a cylindrical rack immersed in an acid-bath pipette-cleaning gizmo filled with aqua regia—a potent mixture of nitric and hydrochloric acids. The acids clean the filter and the pipettes by eating away anything other than the porcelain and glass. A rinse cycle follows, and then the pipettes and candle filters in the vertical rack are allowed to drain and to dry, ready again for use.

One day in late winter 1962, I am setting up my equipment for filtration. I remove the upright candle filter from its drying rack. When I invert it to attach it to the vacuum flask, from the mouth of the candle filter and down the skin of my left inner forearm, from wrist to crook, flows a thick sheet of acid. With horror, I realize that the filter must have been loaded into the dishwasher rack mouth up, so that after it filled with acid, the contents never drained out. The acid on my arm is so concentrated that it is yellow-green and oily. I run screaming to the sink.

Technicians from a nearby lab rush in. I am holding my arm under cold water to rinse off as much of the acid as I can before using the safety solution (to avoid being injured by the additional heat generated by the neutralizing reaction), and they grab the huge plastic carboy of sodium bicarbonate and pour the supersaturated solution of baking soda on my arm. A few drops of the acid from the candle filter have fallen on my white lab skirt, on my shoe, and on the floor. I am astonished that I feel no pain, and I am afraid to look. When finally I can bring myself to glance down at my arm, plastered with sodium bicarbonate, I cannot believe what I see. No sign of any burn at all.

Where the acid has fallen, I have a hole in my skirt and a hole in my shoe. There is even a small hole in the floor.

I have two intact, unblemished arms.

Thank you, Dr. Rosenkrantz. And thank you, God.

Seven

Medical School— Married and Pregnant

September 1962. I am a first-year medical student at Albert Einstein College of Medicine. My husband is an intern in pediatrics at Bellevue. We are living in a basement apartment in the Bronx, around the corner and up the street from Einstein. I am one of seven women in a class of ninety-seven. Two women are married, four are single, and one is a nun.

To follow his graduation from medical school in Cincinnati, hoping to coordinate acceptances in one of the cities, Julie applied for internships and I for admission to medical schools in Boston, New York, and Philadelphia. During the application

process at Harvard Medical School, one of the interviewers—
a woman physician, as it happened—told me that although
I was otherwise qualified, the fact that I was married made it
unlikely that they would accept me. "We are concerned that
married women might get pregnant and drop out," she said to
my face. That's the way it was in 1961.

As a matter of fact, the candor of the Harvard interviewer
was a good step *up* from my experience two years earlier, when
I had applied for admission to the University of Cincinnati
College of Medicine, where Julie, my fiancé at the time, was
a member of the sophomore class. After two academic years
living a distance apart, he and I hoped I'd be admitted to Cincinnati medical school to follow my junior year at Wellesley—
an early start to medical education possible at some medical
schools at that time.

As incredible as it seems to me today, in spite of repeated
requests for some answer, I never received a response from the
medical school. The admissions office simply avoided acting
on my application. We married the following year, I moved
to Cincinnati, and I had to postpone beginning my medical
education until my husband graduated and we could move
back east.

The one thing Julie and I enjoyed while living in Cincinnati were the college basketball games, especially the exciting
state finals between U.C.'s team, which featured the "Big O"
(Oscar Robertson) and rival Ohio State, where Jerry Lucas
and John Havlicek were the stars. We were not fans, however,
of chili parlours and beer, of Kahn's: "the wiener the world

awaited," or of summer opera at the zoo. By the time my husband graduated, we had had enough of "the Queen City," whose newspaper classified employment ads at the time included listings for "colored" and "white," whose politics were Taft-Republican, and whose partisans ripped the Kennedy for President sign from our living room window. I found even Cincinnati's tap water to be unpalatable. It was Ohio River water, treated with so many chemicals that what came out of the faucet had to be something other than one hundred percent water, and had an unpleasant smell to boot.

My work at the research institute was anything but satisfying, close friendships were not in the offing, and with only Julie for company, I found myself increasingly lonely. Newly married, I had to accept the reality that I was, for the most part, unhappy. I ventured the hope that a return to the East Coast, closer to friends and familiar places, would help. The letter informing me that I was wait-listed at Harvard came as no surprise. Cause for celebration were acceptance letters from Albert Einstein College of Medicine, NYU, and several other medical schools willing to take a chance on admitting a married woman. I chose Einstein when Julie chose Bellevue for his internship, and we headed for New York.

We are living on an intern's salary of three hundred dollars per month, so money is very tight, but we can make it. I need a microscope, but I can use my husband's, as well as some of his books. I've got enough scholarships and loans to cover tuition and other books. Classes are barely under way when, in October 1962, the second month of my first year of medical school, after I've been married for two and one-half years and regular with birth control, I know—even before I miss a period—that I am pregnant.

Abortion is illegal but obtainable, if scary. Anyway, I don't want to have an abortion. Even though I'm not so sure about my marriage, it feels right to me, at twenty-three, to be pregnant. In spite of everything, and in the face of having no bloody idea how we will manage, I am glad about this pregnancy. There's no question about it: I know that I want this baby. When I talk Julie into a session with a marriage counselor, the upshot is a recommendation that each of us seek individual therapy. I begin and stick with it for years. He starts and quits. Who knows if therapy would have helped, but at the time we both know that this does not bode well for the marriage.

I find, gratefully, that in spite of our personal problems, I am enjoying medical school. I love studying slides of tissues in histology—magnified images of intricate, patterned cellular structures. Anatomy lectures are fine as well. However, gross anatomy lab—aptly named if you ask me in my first trimester of pregnancy—is somewhat of a problem. The odor of formaldehyde is particularly disgusting when I am suffering with morning sickness. Fortunately, my dissecting partner, Lenny, has plans to become an orthopedic surgeon and is enthusiastic about taking over the dissection. I am happy to accommodate him. On the whole, I am doing very well. I decide that the Harvard interviewer was half, but only half, right. Here I am, a married woman in medical school and, indeed, newly pregnant. However, I am determined to use all my ingenuity to find a way to have this baby, be a good mother, and not drop out.

The challenge will be to raise the funds and to find someone qualified and dependable to take care of the baby while I
am in class. I've had to rely on scholarships, work, and loans
for college and medical school to this point, and I'm not easily
discouraged. My search turns up a book that lists the named
scholarship funds in the United States—hundreds of potential
sources idiosyncratic in their requirements: one with bequests
left "for the benefit of descendants of Daughters of the American Revolution"; one requiring the recipient to be an Eagle
Scout; many with specific or obscure geographic limitations;
and some for which, thankfully, I do qualify. I apply to every one
of these. I am especially hopeful about the American Medical Women's Association, whose offices are right here in New
York City.

The school year moves along. Second semester we begin to
learn psychiatry. Every Friday morning, we have a lecture in
the main lecture hall, followed by a trek over to Bronx Municipal Hospital's inpatient psychiatric unit. For a welcome change,
we are not studying laboratory preparations and cadavers; we
get to see living patients.

Our class is divided into groups of twelve or so, each meeting with a psychiatric preceptor for two hours on the psychiatric ward. My preceptor, Dr. Will Tanenbaum, each week
invites a patient from the psychiatric unit in to speak to him
while we watch and listen. He also gives us a loose-leaf binder
full of reprints of articles and other readings to serve as backup
text for discussions about the patients we will begin to get
to know.

Studying the history of psychoanalysis, I learn that Sigmund

Freud died in 1939, the year I was born. Now, in 1962, the practice of psychoanalysis is, in sophisticated circles in the United States, in its prime. Having grown up in Worcester, Massachusetts, however, my exposure to psychiatry has until now been limited to satisfying a rather bizarre requirement of Wellesley College: that any student requesting recommendation to medical school be interviewed by the school psychiatrist. (I suppose that the premed committee believed it their duty to ascertain whether the rigors of medical education might send a female student over the edge. Or maybe they believed that a woman had to be crazy to want to go to medical school?)

There certainly was a time when referral to the school psychiatrist would have been an appropriate move. During my sophomore year, in the face of Julie's pressure to marry, my mother's wish that I marry him, and my feeling of unreadiness to make a life commitment, I went to talk over my problems with the class dean. Her unhesitating advice to me was: "Don't do what I did. Don't end up an old maid. Marry him!"

Decades later, at my thirty-fifth Wellesley College reunion (my dearest college friend, Linda, never goes, and I've taken myself only to one other), a former dorm-mate and I got to talking about paths taken and paths not taken. Louise told me that when she was in college, she had had dreams of going to medical school and had gone to talk the decision over with the dean. "It will be a financial strain for your family. Give up this idea" was the dean's advice to her. Louise did give it up, to her later regret. I wondered how many other young women the dean "helped."

I had not raised the matter of my commitment to medical school, about which I had no conflict, in my meeting with the dean, and the following year, at the interview required for recommendation by the premed committee, I dutifully met with the school psychiatrist. There he sat, smoking a pipe. I recall only one question he asked: "Name a book you read over the summer." "*Lady Chatterley's Lover,*" I blurted out—a novel that had until recently been banned from American bookstores as scandalously sexually explicit. *Put that in your pipe and smoke it!* Who knows what he thought?

Four years later I do get to know what my psychiatric preceptor, Dr. Tanenbaum, thinks. I also begin to know much more about what I think. Those Friday mornings in the winter and spring of 1963 are among the high points of my life. To have found *a way in,* a means of understanding the ways we cope with the pain of being, an intellectual structure upon which to hang some of the chaos makes my cheeks flush and my heart beat faster. I can't believe that I can someday get paid to understand people and, at the same time, learn to connect more clearly with myself—a life's work that feels like the best of those long conversations with my dear friend Linda. No question about it. This is my calling.

As the year goes on and my pregnancy advances, I wait hopefully for some encouraging word in the way of a prospective grant or loan. I'm beginning to be desperate for the funds we will need for child care, and I come up with the idea of trying to sell the story of my pregnancy to a women's magazine. After I contact several, I'm fortunate to find a receptive audience at *Redbook.* Vivian Cadden, a feature writer who will later become the magazine's editor, agrees to pay some sum of money (I think it was five hundred dollars) for the story of my pregnancy—from the angle of interviews with my husband.

Every four weeks or so, *he* gets to go to lunch at an East Side restaurant with Ms. Cadden to fill her in, from his perspective, on the intimate, pregnancy-related happenings of the month. He distinctly enjoys his part in this. The lunches are delicious, he says, and Ms. Cadden is quite agreeable. I never even meet her. I'm carrying our baby, and he gets the lunches . . . oh well. They pay us and the following year publish the pseudonymous feature, "A Husband's Diary of His Wife's Pregnancy." Julie's sister happens to read the piece and comments to him, "This *Redbook* article sounds a lot like you and Sue." Selling our story was intrusion enough. We never tell our families.

The first year of medical school winds down, and no solution to the baby-care dilemma has presented itself. We do, however, manage a move out of the basement and across the street, to a brighter one-and-a-half-bedroom apartment on the second floor of a large building. Prospects dim when I am finally called for an interview by the American Medical Women's Association to learn from their representative, who is regretful, that they have no available funds.

By mid-July, I am hugely pregnant and running out of hope. The baby is due the third week of August. The first day of classes for my second year of medical school will fall on my twenty-fourth birthday, September 4, 1963—only about seven weeks away—and we have no resources for child care. I don't know how I will be able to continue.

One very hot and humid morning in late July, I receive a

telephone call from a woman who identifies herself as a social worker for the "Adopt-a-Family Association of New York," a Red Feather agency funded by the United Way. The American Medical Women's Association had passed my application along to her. I cannot remember her name, but I do clearly remember her beginning by raising the idea that perhaps I would do well to take a year or so off from school to stay home with the baby. Music. Marriage. I've had all I can take of other people telling me what to do with my life. I interrupt her with a sharpness I think back on with embarrassment but also with pride: "If you don't have funds to help me to go back to school in September, I don't want to talk to you."

The well-meaning woman is quick to assure me that her agency does, indeed, have money to give and suggests kindly that, since I am in my ninth month of pregnancy, perhaps I'd better not travel into the city. She schedules a home visit to discuss my financial needs.

Cleaning help is a budget item for the coming year. Housekeeping assistance has always provided nurture and support—something more than a clean house—for me, something I've known that I need, have made a priority, and for which I will sacrifice. I make no effort to conceal what might be considered to be an indulgence. The social worker arrives for the home visit while the cleaning person who comes a few hours each week is standing on a chair, washing New York City grit off the window blinds.

Remarkably, for each of the next three years, the Adopt-a-Family Association of New York will grant the twenty-six hundred dollars needed to pay Honey, the kind, warm, dependable, low-key mother of two grown sons who answers our ad and comes as needed to take care of Jennifer until I graduate and we move to Boston. Truth be told, there are times when I feel as though Honey is taking care of me. On a couple of occasions, while Julie is on call or away, the baby and I both spend the night with Honey and her family in their comfortable home in suburban Yonkers.

When I think back on those times, sometimes I wonder whether the Adopt-a-Family Association actually existed. I never saw its office. I met the social worker only that one time. If ever I had needed an angel, I had been sent one.

This bit of writing in William H. Murray's *The Scottish Himalayan Expedition* (1951) sings out with a grace and rhythm unlike the rest of Murray's language:

> *The moment one definitely commits oneself, then Providence moves too. All sorts of things occur to help one that would never otherwise have occurred. A whole stream of events issues from the decision, raising in one's favour all manner of unforeseen incidents and meetings and material assistance which no man could have dreamed would come his way.*

"Then Providence moves too . . ." Sometimes, anyway. Thankfully for me in 1963, Providence moved for certain.

Eight

Of Guilt
and Wonder

When *I think back on the events of spring and early sum-*mer 1964, now forty years past, a confusion of feelings, strong as ever, floods in. The feelings? Guilt, relief, fear, wonder, gratitude, and still, wonder . . .

It happens this way. In the second semester of my second year of medical school, I am just about managing to mother my beloved nine-month-old daughter while cramming to learn pharmacology, biostatistics, clinical pathology, parasitology—the last of the preclinical sciences—and my period is late. Just a couple of days late, but it's usually like clockwork. No simple trip to the drugstore for a home pregnancy test in those days; I'll have to wait weeks for laboratory confirmation. But from the way my body feels, I'm certain.

And I am worried. Unlike my first pregnancy, which, while unplanned and clearly coming at a difficult time, I wanted, this time I am having another experience altogether. Yes, it would be very difficult to stretch myself to mother another child—but somehow that's not the defining matter. I can't say exactly *what* is frightening me, but I know that I want to end this pregnancy, and urgently. Unaccountably, I couldn't possibly be less conflicted about what would normally be a very difficult decision. And I know that finding a safe way to end it will not be a simple matter at all.

Abortions are still illegal in the United States. Except, that is, in instances of "medical necessity"—to save the life of the mother, for example, or if the mother contracts German measles during the first three months of pregnancy. Serious birth defects are known to be caused by infection, during the first trimester, with the rubella virus, the one that causes German measles.

The week my period doesn't come around, what do you know? One of my female lab partners comes down with German measles. When I mention this to my husband, who is doing his residency in pediatrics, he reports that there's an epidemic of the virus here in the Bronx. He's good with the facts. I'm alone with the rest.

It's nearly spring vacation, and I'm planning to take our baby to visit my parents in Worcester. The unholy idea comes to me of a way I can try to obtain a legal abortion. Do I dare to go to a gynecologist in Worcester *and tell him that I have just recovered from German measles and believe that I am pregnant?*

I do.

The well-recommended doctor I go to see listens to my story, examines me, and says that we have a dilemma. He says that if, in fact, I am pregnant, I *must* have a D&C. But then he goes on to tell me that, since it is actually too early to confirm that I am pregnant, he would prefer to wait. I explain to him (at least this is the truth) that I have the week off and must then get back for midterm exams at medical school, and I plead with him to do the procedure right away. When he agrees to admit me to the hospital the next day, I am immensely relieved, but I also feel guilty—not for choosing to end this pregnancy (if, in fact, I really am pregnant)—but for lying.

One overnight in the hospital and I am back home at my parents'. I've got an appointment at the end of the week for a post-op checkup with the gynecologist. That day, in his consulting room, he looks over the pathology report of the tissue removed at the D&C and says to me, "Well, you definitely were pregnant. And it's a good thing we did the surgery. The virus you had certainly did a lot of damage. The implant was hydropic." I have never before heard that term, *hydropic*. He goes on to explain that the rubella virus had completely destroyed the developing embryo, and that if I hadn't had the D&C, I would have begun to miscarry within a couple of weeks. He adds that I might have had to have a D&C then. I am confused beyond imagining. *How can this be? I know, even if he doesn't, that I have* not *had German measles.*

The weekend comes, and we drive back to the Bronx. I am still experiencing a mix of puzzlement, relief, and guilt when, on Monday, I break out in a rash. Can I believe it? German measles. The virus must have been in my body, incubating for its standard two to three weeks. No wonder the implant was hydropic. Have I lied, or have I been prescient? Of course I shall never know.

The twilight zone widens in a scary way a couple of days later, when the rash is just about gone but I notice a very dark bruise on the inside of my right upper arm. This appears really to be more than a bruise. It is a black spot. I have had no injury, and I have no idea at all how to account for the ominous-looking lesion. When I show it to my husband, he asks to look at the underside of my tongue. Then he gently pulls down and inspects the insides of my lower eyelids. Tiny red dots, pinpoint hemorrhages called petechiae (pet-TEE-key-eye), show up in both places. I look in the mirror and am frightened when I see them for myself. What I've learned about this kind of bleeding is that it means my body's clotting mechanisms are not normal, something that I know can happen in leukemia and in other very serious illnesses.

My husband has some partially reassuring information. He thinks what I've got is something he's been seeing recently on the pediatric ward, where he has admitted several children with similar symptoms—all of them just recovering from German measles. He suspects that, like them, I have developed something called ITP—idiopathic thrombocytopenic purpura—not a cancer but an autoimmune illness triggered by the body's response to fighting off the rubella virus. He tells me that ITP is most usually a one-time illness that can be treated with steroids until it runs its course. Julie has a lancet and some slides in his medical bag, and I let him prick my finger and make a slide, which he runs over to the hospital lab to look at under the microscope.

He's back quickly with the verdict: I've got ITP, and I've got it bad. The slide showed no sign of any platelets, the tiny cell fragments that are a key clotting factor and of which normally we have hundreds of thousands per cubic millimeter of blood. Having no platelets, I have a potentially life-threatening condition, where coughing can cause a stroke, and where brushing my teeth could induce a hemorrhage. I've got to be in a hospital, and right away. We head out for Columbia Presbyterian, in Manhattan, where I am admitted on the spot.

When the doctors ask the details of my recent medical history, of course I tell them everything, including the fact that I had a D&C the previous week, was found to be pregnant, and had a hydropic embryo. I leave out the detail about having lied. I am relieved when nobody asks. One of them does say, "Well, it's a good thing you had that procedure when you did, because if you had remained pregnant, you would certainly have had a spontaneous abortion, and with no platelets, I'm not sure we could have stopped the bleeding."

I realize that I might well owe my life to the unusually clear and unconflicted conviction I had not to continue this pregnancy, to the lie I chose to tell in order to terminate it, and to the physician who stretched the rules by performing what he believed to be—and, eerily, *what turned out to be*—a legal abortion before I could be proven definitely to be pregnant.

I don't think about this experience very often. But when I do, even after forty years, those feelings flood in: guilt, relief, fear, wonder, gratitude, and still, wonder . . .

Nine

What I Owe
to Dr. F.

June 1964. I've had a rocky course with ITP, I'm still on steroids, and I've made it through the first two years of medical school, the preclinical years. Jennifer is a beautiful, chubby ten-month-old, pulling herself up to stand by holding on to our bookcases, then happily knocking the books, one by one, to the floor. Julie and I are sharing the wonders of parenthood, but other than that, our marriage is a thin connection. I continue in therapy, which feels like a veritable lifeline, and I am surer than ever that I want to be a psychiatrist. When third-year schedules are posted, I learn that my first clinical rotation will be six weeks on the pediatric floor at Montefiore Hospital in the Bronx.

I have no idea what I am in for.

My first day on Pediatrics begins with early-morning rounds, where I follow the interns and residents from bed to bed while they review each medical chart, look at lab reports and test results, examine the patient, discuss the illness, consider treatment options, and plan the medical interventions for the coming day. Here on Pediatrics, the beds are cribs, and the patients, mostly, are toddlers. Very, very sick toddlers. Of the fifteen or so children I meet, several have brain tumors, and others are suffering from advanced stages of leukemia. It's hard for me not to think of my own beautiful, healthy baby, and I pray that she continue to be spared any such horrible fate.

The tasks assigned to the two of us medical students on this particular rotation include drawing blood for lab tests. In the past we have practiced drawing blood on one another. It's not been pleasant, but it's not been terrible. We had to learn, after all. But drawing blood from a more or less cooperative adult is a different matter altogether from drawing blood from a very sick, screaming child.

Absolutely the worst, though, is the fact that babies and small children have very, very small veins. I am not prepared for the ways in which blood sometimes must be drawn. From infants, it is sometimes drawn from veins in their scalp. Sometimes, from older children, it is drawn from the jugular vein in the neck. I can't bear it. I simply can't bear it. I can't even bear to write about it.

I'm barely managing to hold myself together when, one night when I am on call, a two-year-old girl with blond curls is admitted from the emergency room. It seems that she had a cold but was otherwise fine until today, when suddenly she began to have serious trouble breathing. The pediatric resident tells me that the child now has developed epiglottitis—an inflammation of the epiglottis, the flap that covers the voice box. Her epiglottis is so swollen that it is obstructing her airway. This is an emergency, and the only hope is a tracheotomy.

All I can remember after that is a crowd of pediatricians and nurses clustered around the little body, performing the procedure to try to save this little girl's life. Tragically, it is to no avail. Later in the night, she dies.

Maybe the steroids I've been taking for three months have taken their toll on my emotional reserves, but I am ready to crack. I cannot manage any more of this pediatric rotation. The following day, I go to speak to the head of the inpatient Department of Pediatrics. I don't remember his name, except that it began with the letter F, but I will never forget his help. I tell him that I think that maybe I have to quit medical school. Dr. F. listens to me, patiently, then says, "Listen. Take some time off. You don't have to quit. You're doing fine learning what you need to know about pediatrics. When you're ready, come back, but don't do any procedures you aren't comfortable with."

What a decent man! I did take several days off, and when I returned, somehow I got through the required couple of weeks with nothing in my hands more intrusive than a stethoscope.

During subsequent clinical rotations, I found, thankfully,

that I was not similarly squeamish in doing what was required for sick adult patients. I'll never know what part the steroids might have played in my vulnerability to the pediatric crisis. I am sure that being a mother to my own baby together with my memories of having been on the receiving end of frightening medical treatments during my early childhood contributed significantly to my coming so close to the brink of quitting. If Dr. F. had been a man of different character or politics, less compassionate, less well disposed to women in medicine . . .

I don't like to think about what might have happened.

Ten

Transitions

*J*uly 1965. *Julie has completed his pediatric residency program.*
This is my last year of medical school, and I've got another six
months of various clinical rotations at Einstein before a final
half-year elective at a medical center of my choice. Jennifer
is almost two and thriving. Although our marriage is not, we
make the best plan we can: we will move to Boston, a city we
both love and a place where we enjoyed many happy times the
first years we were dating. My husband arranges to take over a
general pediatric practice from a physician who is leaving to
subspecialize in pediatric allergy. Spending weekdays apart for

the first six months may not be a bad idea. We'll find an apartment in a Boston suburb for Julie, and the baby and I will continue here as we are. Jenni can sleep at Honey's when I have to be on call, and I'll take the air shuttle to Boston with her to be with Julie most weekends. So that is what we do from July through December.

When it's time for the full move to Boston, Julie's practice is going well enough that we can afford to hire Mayflower Van Lines to pack up the apartment as well as to move everything. Like locusts systematically eating their way through vegetation, the moving men pack their way through our Bronx apartment. Everything gets wrapped and boxed. Half a piece of apple pie on a plate on the coffee table? Wrapped in corrugated cardboard and packed. I swear.

A stroke of good fortune: my mother's friend Bette is available to take care of Jennifer while I'm at work. When I myself was small, too infrequently, Bette took care of me. She was warm, calm, and gave wonderful back rubs. Jenni will miss Honey, and there's no help for that, but I am comforted with the prospect that she will come to love Bette, too. I'm certain that having Bette around will be a good thing for me, as well.

In Boston, before we have even unpacked, I find myself in marathon mode working my way through the psychiatric units of several of Harvard's teaching hospitals. I will spend a month or two in sequence at McLean Hospital, Massachusetts Mental Health Center, and Beth Israel Hospital—an intensive elective for the five months leading up to graduation. I'm in the flow of learning the work of psychiatry, and I am loving it.

McLean Hospital, an elite and very expensive private mental hospital in Belmont, west of Cambridge, is my first assignment. The campus of rolling greens and stone buildings looks something like Wellesley College, but there most of the similarity ends. Appleton House, where I am based, is the only unlocked unit, a residence for the patients considered well enough to come and go independent of escort, responsible to report their whereabouts to staff.

My first day, I sit in on rounds with the psychiatrist in charge at the time, Dr. M. During this oddly formal and casual ritual that takes place in Appleton's living room, one at a time the patients come in to talk to Dr. M. A staff nurse, charts at the ready and order book in her lap, makes notes. I learn that treatment of patients at McLean operates on the basis of a "therapist/administrator split," which translates to each patient's having not one, but *two* psychiatrists: one responsible for conducting psychotherapy, the other in charge of making administrative decisions—such as with which degree of "privileges" to move about the hospital unaccompanied the patient may be entrusted. The idea behind this apparent division of labor is to foster the patient-therapist alliance: the patient is supposed to feel free to confide fully in the therapist without risking loss of privileges, the domain of the administrator-psychiatrist. When I hear this, I am certain that the absurdity of this construct cannot be lost on the patients. Imagine a patient telling his therapist anything consequential in the way of risk that the therapist would withhold from the administrator? Not bloody likely.

I don't get to see much of this tangle at Appleton House,

though, populated as it is with patients who have convinced both their therapists and their administrators that they don't need much supervision. Virtually all of them have been in the hospital for months, some for years, many having graduated to Appleton from the locked units. If I think I'm going to learn much at rounds about what in the world ever brought them to McLean, I've got another think coming. What I do learn goes something like this:

PATIENT A.: My father wants me to accompany him on a trip to Martinique for a couple of weeks.

DR. M.: If you want to go, why not? It will be a lot less expensive for you than staying here—that's for sure.

Little by little, I learn that McLean does not reflect much of the world that most of us inhabit. At baseline, it costs a fortune. Wealthy patients commonly stay a year or more. Patients with insurance coverage remain until their benefits run out, at which point they are either discharged or transferred to a state hospital.

That the professional staff at McLean includes a roster of some of Boston's most highly regarded psychiatrists, that the physical facility is top-notch and the nursing staff competent is outweighed, in my opinion, by the policy that, on admission, patients, even those who are not known to be suicidal, are routinely stripped of freedom and responsibility for themselves and are expected to remain in the hospital for months to years. When I continue the elective psychiatric clerkship the following month at Massachusetts Mental Health Center, I am impressed to find this small state hospital to have an extraordinarily fine staff and to be, with regard to patient autonomy and term of hospitalization, the polar opposite of McLean. Given the importance that respect for individual self-determination holds for me, I prefer the philosophy of treatment of the publicly funded hospital by far.

Mass Mental (the epithet is both short and fitting) consists of one shabby three-story longish brick building in a busy Boston neighborhood where, in 1966, three-decker wood houses still manage a toehold amid the expanding medical centers of the Brigham, the Deaconess, and Children's hospitals. One such formerly residential building across the street from Mass Mental has been appropriated as-is for a couple of offices and a meeting place for the group-therapy training program. In the main building, a small troop of men with ladders, paint cans, and brushes perpetually work their way through the hospital interior, upstairs and down, from one end to the other, trying to paint the place clean. Like the painters on the Brooklyn Bridge, as soon as they get to one end, they have to begin again at the other.

There are no locked doors at Mass Mental. Not one. Of course, some of the patients need close supervision—those who are psychotic and confused, those at risk of suicide—but watch is kept by a staff member sitting alongside the open door of each inpatient unit, through which most of the patients and staff freely come and go. An atmosphere of respect for autonomy prevails. Together Dr. Elvin Semrad, who is head of residency training, and Dr. Jack Ewalt, the hospital chief administrator, have created a uniquely sane mental hospital and an extraordinary, world-class psychiatric teaching program.

In radical contrast with the policy at McLean, one of Dr. Semrad's basic tenets is:

> *When you use a hospital for any more than riding over a crisis and attaching to a therapist, then you're not running a hospital, you're running a hotel.*

As a medical student, I am assigned to inpatient Service Three, where, in consultation with the residents to whom they are regularly assigned, I share in the treatment of a couple of patients. Integrated into the busy life of the unit, I attend the daily community meetings of all the patients and staff and the daily teaching conferences as well. Here Dr. Semrad or another senior staff member or visiting psychiatrist meets with the psychiatric residents-in-training, medical students, social workers, social-work students, psychology interns, divinity students, and occupational-therapy students (Mass Mental is surely a teaching hospital) to be "presented a patient." Following a format that includes *history of chief complaint* (how the patient came to be admitted to the hospital), *relevant family history, medical history,* and *mental status,* the resident provides information and formulates particular questions to prepare the teacher for conducting an interview with the patient in the presence of the group. In Dr. Semrad's teaching conferences, on completion of the interview, Semrad always respectfully asks the patient, "May I have your permission to talk to your doctor about your problem?"

I soon find that experienced psychiatrists and trainees alike look forward to the conferences he chairs as the high point of the week. There we see his patience, warmth, respect for others, and deep commitment to the necessity for people to make their own decisions. With gentle firmness, in his interviews with patients, Semrad demonstrates an extraordinary ability to expose the heart of many a central but elusive matter. He can even get the most psychotic, the craziest patients to settle down and talk to him. Semrad's focus is most often on whatever emotional pain the patient has been trying not to have to feel. He stresses the importance of helping our patients to acknowledge and grieve their losses adequately in order to go on.

It is clear that Semrad believes in the possibilities of man and in the primacy of feeling. He recognizes the common use of self-deception as an avoidance of pain. He believes in the importance of being able to acknowledge reality, grapple with it and bear it, and put it into perspective in order to deal with life and to grow. He has a special ability to simplify the complex, to recognize, identify, and describe the feelings common to people, and to communicate this in his clinical work and teaching.

My experience at Mass Mental in 1966 is alive, alive, alive, and I love it. Too quickly the two months pass, but by happy chance, the third hospital in my rotation, Beth Israel, a general hospital with one psychiatric floor, is just a few blocks away. I manage to convince the psychiatrists who have been supervising my work at Mass Mental to continue so that I will be allowed to go on meeting with my patients, and I shuttle back and forth for the last month of the elective, excited to be learning psychotherapy.

In June, Julie, Jennifer (who is nearly three), and I, along with my parents and Bette, drive to New York for my graduation. At the time, we don't know that this will be the last point of celebration in our marriage. The crisis comes soon after we return to Boston, when Julie proposes that, for the coming year, we move to a quieter location closer to his practice. Initially, this seems like a good idea, and quite soon we find a suitable suburban house available to rent. However, when I actually sit with the lease in hand to commit to one more year of living together, I find that I cannot bring myself to pick up the pen.

This is the end of my marriage.

We decide that I will remain in what has been our apartment with Jennifer and, within a couple of weeks, when I begin to serve my internship, Julie will find a place of his own. One natural transition is in the offing—he will return to spend the many nights and weekends with Jenni that I am on call.

I will certainly be away from Jennifer far more than I want to, and clearly more than is good for her and me. This is a heavy piece. But in the face of my personal confusion of feelings, I find that for the most part I welcome the busyness. I could definitely do with more sleep, though. Internship schedules are demanding to the point of craziness. I will be working every day from eight A.M. to five P.M., and will have to remain to staff the hospital all night every other night, as well as every other weekend. A sample workweek: Monday morning until Tuesday evening, Wednesday morning until Thursday evening, and all day Friday. Weekend call duty: Saturday morning through Monday evening, every other week. Oftentimes up all night. Grueling, absolutely grueling.

My first internship assignment is the emergency room. Fresh from the experience of the psychiatric elective, I find myself stressed to the limits by the physical and emotional pain flooding in through the E.R. doors and cresting high. In psychiatric clerkship, I had been developing skills at connecting with a patient's experience, learning how to help carry the burden of pain while keeping the boundaries clear. Now, as a medical intern, I realize that if I am going to make it through the year I will have to find a way to detach, to a considerable degree, from my patients' experiences. Struggling to integrate empathy and detachment, I get to some survivable level and carry on.

A few patients, in particular, push the limits of this balance. Of the hundreds I treat this challenging year, they are among the few who, four decades later, I specifically remember. One is a delicate middle-aged woman dying from metastatic ovarian cancer. My heart breaks every time I see her. Her courage, grace, and will to live remind me of my beloved aunt Bess, whose extended struggle with breast cancer ended painfully just a few months earlier.

Another is a teenage Greek girl who was hit by a car, suffered a concussion, and is brought in to the emergency room unconscious. Her relatives tell me that she does not speak one word of English. Since my knowledge of Greek is limited to *souvlaki* and *Phi Beta Kappa*, I ask her family for help, and scribble transliterations of the words for "Do you have pain?" (*Ponai?*) and "Are you thirsty?" (*Thebsas?*) on her pillow. In order to monitor her emergence to consciousness, every fifteen minutes through the night I whisper in her ear: *Maria, ponai? Maria, thebsas?* She wakes, I am relieved, and I will always remember her—and these Greek words.

To the extent that the workload permits, we interns become friends. We certainly have common interests. Five of the eight of us have plans to specialize in psychiatry. It turns out, in fact, that three of us are applying, as a first choice, to the residency program at Mass Mental. One of the group, Mike Weiner, likes to cook. There is a grill outside the nurses' residence, and a couple of times during the summer Mike comes to work with chicken marinating in a bucket in the trunk of his car. It's a wonder we don't get salmonella poisoning. Late in the year there is one inconvenient physical calamity consequential to food preparation. As dessert for a communal meal, I make crème caramel. Swirling molten sugar to coat the custard cups, I spill a drop—hotter than hot—between my fingers. The skin blisters. Now scrubbing and gloving up to assist at surgery is out of the question, and we have to schedule some complicated trading off of surgical duty for the weeks until my fingers heal.

One day in midwinter, we receive our residency matchups. I've figured that if none of us are accepted for training at Mass Mental, we'll commiserate; if one of us gets to go, we can celebrate; but if two are chosen and one left out, it will be really tough. Against the odds, good news comes for all three of us, and the celebration is a full one.

Most of the work we get to do this year can be done by any competent intern, but there is one remarkable experience where my particular contribution is key. It happens in late winter, when a thirty-five-year-old woman is brought to the emergency room by ambulance. Her family doctor has just phoned in to alert us that she is having a cerebral hemorrhage, a kind of stroke. On arrival, she is unable to speak, so her husband provides the medical history: nausea, vomiting, headache, and stiff neck. Classic for an intracranial bleed—a medical emergency that can result in pressure-related brain damage.

The resident notifies the operating room that we are sending a patient up for a burr-hole procedure (small holes to be drilled through the bones of her skull), a crude but effective way to relieve dangerously high pressure. While preparations are under way, I continue to gather further details of the history of the woman's illness from her husband. When I learn that for treatment of her first symptom, nausea, her doctor had prescribed Compazine, a bell goes off. I know that Compazine is chemically related to Thorazine, which is a potent tranquilizer used to treat psychosis. During my elective in psychiatry, I learned that Thorazine can cause potentially bizarre side effects that mimic Parkinson's disease or stroke. And I know that epinephrine is a kind of antidote for such crises.

In the heat of preparations for sending the patient to the O.R., when I suggest to the resident that we give the patient some intravenous epinephrine, he brushes me off. I persist, and at the last minute, he allows that, okay, I can try it. I inject the epinephrine, *and the patient's symptoms clear up before our eyes.* Her surgery is cancelled, and the job falls to me to stay with her through the night to regulate the epinephrine intravenous drip. When it slows down too much, the patient gets stiff again. When it runs too fast, her heart races. By morning, the worst is over, her symptoms are gone, her skull is intact, and I am happy and proud—if exhausted. So it comes to pass that the recognition I receive the following week at medical grand rounds is for my application of something I learned in psychiatry.

A few months later, the last night I spend on call during my internship, I am already unconsciously shifting gears to open my heart to psychiatric patients once again. At about three o'clock in the morning, the telephone rings in the on-call room with a request that I come to the floor to "pronounce" a patient. This means that I am to examine a person who has died, confirm that the patient has expired, write the findings in the chart, and notify the private physician and next of kin. It is a procedure I have performed several times this hard year. Tonight the patient I have been called to see is an old woman who has been on the ward for several weeks, is known to have been letting go of life, and has no private physician or kin to notify.

When I get to the patient, whom the nurse has of course already examined and found to be dead, I carry out the routine protocol. I shine a light at the pupils of her eyes to confirm that they are dilated and do not contract. I put a stethoscope to her chest to confirm that she is not breathing and has no heartbeat, and I go to the nursing station and write the note in the chart. Then I make my way back to the on-call room.

When I sit down on the bed, detachment fails me. The sadness of the end of a life and the reality of my part in the stark medically routine ceremony of closure to this woman's life wash over me, and I am startled by a thought:

What if she isn't really dead?

Pulled by a compulsion to return to the ward to examine the patient again, I go back. I don't even try to explain to the nurse what I am doing. The light. The stethoscope. The old woman is still dead. But I am more alive, connected once again to a full experience of existential pain.

I am ready to become a psychiatrist.

Eleven

Psychiatric
Residency

On *July 1, 1967, I find that I am the only woman in a* psychiatric residency group of twenty-five. I am also the recently divorced mother of a three-year-old who needs as much loving attention as I can possibly give. We've survived the internship year, and the prospects here are clearly better. There are so many residents at Mass Mental that the call schedule is very light—maybe one night a month or so, and no full weekend duty. The regular workload will be substantial, but I can make it a priority, if I take absolutely no breaks, to leave every day by six to get home to Jenni.

To make it in to this program, each of us has managed to

pass muster with the no-nonsense hospital administrator, Dr. Jack Ewalt, and with the director of residency training, Dr. Elvin Semrad, whose inspiring teaching during my fourth-year medical school elective had played a significant part in my choice of residency. In 1967, Semrad is a middle-aged, over-weight, pipe-smoking, slow-talking gentleman from the Plains who wears white socks with black leather shoes and who likes to refer to himself as "just a hayseed from Nebraska." His self-abnegation fools none of us. Semrad's genius is legend. He has a way of understanding life and living, a way of getting to the bottom of what drives people crazy that provides a unique and immeasurably valuable foundation for the work of psychiatry. It is pretty damned useful in living our own lives, for that matter.

In Dr. Semrad's homespun language:

The first year, the experience and learning grows from the seat of your pants. The patient is the only textbook we require.

As a psychiatrist, your job is to help the patient stand his pain, and this is directly contrary to the rest of the medical profession.

Laymen often think that the best way to deal with any difficult situation is not to deal with it—to forget it. But you and I have the experience that the only way you can forget is to remember.

A man's either scared, mad, or sad. If he's talking about anything else, he's being superficial.

Symptoms are solutions. Think about the purpose of the symptom: what does the symptom do for the person?

Normality is essentially a function of where, with whom, and when. Anything is all right, so long as it is at the right time, in the right place, and with the right person.

Falling in love is the only socially acceptable psychosis.

We learn early on that psychotherapy is the work of helping our patients to identify and acknowledge painful feelings, to bear them, and, finally, to put them into perspective. This is a mental hospital, and naturally many of our patients are pretty strung-out. One of the first things I am taught is never to put myself between a patient and the door to my office—unless I want to risk being clobbered if the patient's anxiety impels him or her to bolt.

Mass Mental's physical plant is pretty old and, actually, shabby. The room I am assigned as an office has a few special features. It is larger than most, but that's because it was formerly a bathroom. The door has a half panel of frosted glass, and the walls are green tile. A clunky wooden desk is pushed as close as it can get to a tiled wall to which irregular crags of soapstone adhere where sinks were once attached. The most distinctive feature of the room is the floor, which slopes down slightly toward a drain hole in the center. *Hmmmmm. Handy in case I want to hose down the room.*

I do what I can with this primitive space. On the largest

wall, some prior occupant has rigged a canvas covering, to which I manage to pin paper posters. I cover the drain hole and most of the floor with a blue rug and find a plant that can live without natural light. And I make certain to put the patient's chair closest to the door.

Mass Mental has four inpatient units, including one known as the Day Hospital, to which six other residents and I have been assigned. Our patients go home at night in the company of a family member or friend who has consented to the arrangement, but otherwise meet no different criteria for hospitalization than do patients on the day-and-night inpatient services.

A fundamental of Semrad's philosophy of training—commitment to well-supervised long-term psychotherapy—carries through to a unique policy of the teaching program: once a patient is assigned on admission to a psychiatric resident, that assignment is, for the life of the residency experience, "forever." What this means is that when one of my patients is discharged from the hospital, I am to follow the patient on an outpatient basis as long as the patient needs therapy and is willing to come. Additionally, during my years at Mass Mental, if a patient I have ever treated needs readmission, I am to be the psychiatrist assigned.

All three years of my psychiatric residency are blessed and burdened with hours and hours of supervision—six to eight hours per week. Many of the supervisors require process notes— notes made after a therapy session that recap the dialogue of the session, preferably word for word, and with as much detail, accuracy, and honesty as possible. Note taking during the interview is discouraged, a potential distraction both to me and to the patient. The idea is for me to be *in* the experience while observing it. After a few months of tedious process-note making after the fact, I find that, during supervision, I am not relying on my notes at all. The discipline of attention in anticipation of making the notes has developed my ability both to participate and to remember the content and flow of the dialogue, skills fundamental to the work of therapy.

As a first-year resident, no matter that I am eager to begin, in Semrad's words, *to investigate, investigate, investigate*, to try to understand, and to make notes for supervision, confoundingly it happens early on that two of my patients simply won't talk. The first is a man in his late thirties who lives with his mother. She has brought him to the hospital because, that morning, he shot his toothbrush. With a gun. She tells the social worker that her son has recently had an unpleasant experience at the dentist. Her son also has a thick medical chart and a diagnosis of chronic schizophrenia. On this occasion I learn that when reason dictates, a Day Hospital patient can be "guested" overnight on one of the other inpatient units.

The chief resident helpfully advises that in my daily meetings with the patient I keep my office door open. I'm not sure whether the reason for this is to offer no obstacle in case the patient wants to split and run back to the day room or to make it possible for the staff to keep an eye and an ear on the two of us. Either way, I keep the door open. In the same spirit, the chief suggests that I limit his psychotherapy sessions to ten minutes apiece.

Psychotherapy? Well, I try. Gently, you may believe, I ask

questions. The patient just sits. He seems to be thinking about *something*, but he's not talking. Truthfully, I'm not sure which of us is more relieved when the ten minutes are up. We don't have to endure this odd ritual for long, though, because after the patient spends just a few nights in the hospital, his mother wants to have him home. In fact, he goes home for good a couple of mercifully uneventful weeks later, when the social worker reports that, to his mother's satisfaction, her son is back to his old self and will we please discharge him?

My second absolute failure at engaging a patient spans a period of several months and teaches me something critical about brain chemistry and mental illness. Psychoanalytically oriented psychotherapy is my primary interest, a focus well served in this residency program. But Mass Mental is also at the vanguard of adjunctive approaches to mental illness. In a three-decker across the street, Dr. Joseph Schildkraut is doing groundbreaking research on neurochemistry and depression, and on the top floor of the main building, the Clinical Research Center (the CRC) has just begun a placebo-controlled, double-blind study on the effectiveness of two potent and relatively new antipsychotic drugs, Mellaril and Haldol, in the treatment of acute schizophrenia. Fate has it that I am one of seven first-year residents assigned to staff both the Day Hospital and the CRC.

My first CRC patient is Caroline, a young married woman in her early twenties, who was brought to the hospital because, a few days after she gave birth to her first child, she began behaving in a strange way. Actually, she stopped behaving at all.

She . . . just . . . stopped. Caroline no longer talks and seems unaware of herself and of what is happening around her. She moves slowly, looking blank. She does not even use the toilet. When I first see her she is mute, she drools, her long blond hair hangs unkempt, and she smells awful.

At the time, like Semrad, I am not a fan of medication. But I am resigned that, according to the CRC protocol, Caroline will be assigned at random to one of the two antipsychotic medications or a placebo. Neither I nor anyone else on the staff will know what she is receiving. As a CRC therapist, I am permitted to choose the "number of units" of the "medication" I want my patient to receive. If, after several weeks on a given protocol, the patient does not respond, I am permitted to request a change to one of the other of the three options. Even then, I cannot know what the patient is given. I begin by prescribing for Caroline the lowest allowable dose of whatever she has been randomly assigned—privately hoping that it is the placebo. Caroline is clearly in serious trouble, but considering that she was apparently okay until the birth of her baby, I am hopeful that well-supervised psychotherapy and attentive nursing care will restore her to herself and to her baby girl.

And so we begin. Each day we meet for an hour's "psychotherapy," during which Caroline sits blankly and does not talk. Unlike the toothbrush shooter, she does not appear even to be thinking about anything. Everything about her seems to be disorganized—even her brain. Of concern is not only the patient but also her baby—in the care of another family member, but without its mother. In the face of this crisis I cannot help but decide rather quickly that resistance to prescribing psychotropic drugs is absurd, and as soon as I can, I begin increasing the "units" of whatever medication she is receiving. I raise the dose regularly—to the maximum allowed—and, with a growing lack of confidence and increasing unease, continue daily "psychotherapy." Zilch. Caroline remains unreachable. Her fingernails get longer and dirtier. In the face of her showing no sign of improvement, I find myself hoping that she has been receiving the placebo, but for another reason entirely— for the chance that she will benefit from an active drug. As soon as is permitted, I request a switch to another option in the drug protocol.

Within a couple of days, to everyone's great relief, Caroline begins to come back to life. I look forward, finally, to getting to know her. However, in our daily sessions, while she is present and pleasant, Caroline still does not have much to say. Otherwise, her recovery proceeds steadily, she begins to connect with her baby on visits, and within several weeks she is ready to go home. We schedule outpatient sessions, and Caroline comes in dutifully. She says she's fine, life is okay, but no matter how patiently I try, nothing turns up really to work with. Caroline is not self-reflective, has little interest in the world of ideas, and has less curiosity about herself and others than do most small children.

At the time, etched large in the design of a mirror in a Boston subway station are these words:

Each observation you make changes you.

My friend Allie, with whom I used to play chamber music, took a photograph of that mirror, which of course shows her shooting the picture (and which she had to reverse in printing so that the words could be read). Still today I have a grainy enlargement of the image mounted on the inside of my coat-closet door. I get a pulse of pleasure each time I look at it, an affirmation of the confoundingly complex and, to me, fascinating reality that neurochemistry impacts *and is impacted upon* by everything we think and feel and with which we come in contact—including, for many people, the work of psychotherapy. Unfortunately, my patient Caroline is not one for making, or listening to, observations. After a couple of months my supervisor and I have to accept it: Caroline is not one for psychotherapy.

I learn from Caroline that sometimes drugs are the only option. To prescribe drugs when a patient's brain chemistry is out of whack and where the beneficial effects clearly outweigh the costs is basic medical practice. But I learn also that the pharmaceutical manipulation of brain chemistry holds no compelling interest for me. I find stimulation and satisfaction with those patients who, whether taking psychotropic medications or not, *do* sit and talk to me to engage in the work of facing the truth of their thoughts and feelings.

Drugs change brain chemistry, can have subtle to devastating side effects, and don't do much for the soul. For those who can be engaged, skillful psychotherapy also changes brain chemistry and offers a trade-off of the pain of neurotic and psychotic symptoms for the pain and pleasure of existential reality. Semrad used to say:

I've never seen a group that is more hopeful or willing to believe in magic than the endocrine people. They think if they can just find the right juice, life will be an endless pleasure.

We're in an era where treatment is not popular. We're in a manipulation era. [This, in the 1960s!]

The 1960s is a transitional time in psychiatry. The psychoanalytic movement is at its peak, neuropsychiatry is at its beginnings, and a political slant on psychiatry has a popular voice in the writings of the British psychiatrist R. D. Laing (*The Politics of Experience* and *The Divided Self*) and an American psychiatrist, Thomas Szasz (*The Myth of Mental Illness*), each in his own way declaring that psychopathology is generated by the ills of society and/or interpersonal relationships, and that social change and/or psychoanalytically oriented psychotherapy is what is needed.

In 1968, R. D. Laing comes to Boston to speak at Brandeis, as well as at one of our regular Wednesday noon guest conferences at Mass Mental. A handsome, charismatic man with a strong Scottish brogue, Laing draws such a crowd that, even allowing for standees, we cannot fit into the chapel where, Mass Mental having no auditorium as such, guest conferences are generally held. The fallback is the gymnasium. This huge space becomes packed as well.

When Laing begins to speak, I am reminded at first of a recent talk by MIT's linguistic expert, Noam Chomsky. The common element is that I cannot understand a word. The difficulty here, though, is not one of lucidity, and once I accustom myself to Laing's brogue, I take in his observation—one that will serve constructively throughout my years of practice—that psychiatric disorders and symptoms can be understood as attempts on the part of a person to deal with inevitable existential uncertainty. Semrad has said: *Symptoms are solutions*. Laing extends this to an observation that *symptoms are solutions that work by creating an illusion of certainty about something.*

Take, for example, a woman who is racked with worry that something terrible will happen. If her concern is severe, she may qualify for the label of *phobic*. Let's say she is afraid to fly on a plane. If she does travel by air, she will suffer anxiety in anticipation and during the flight, but once she disembarks the plane: *Whew, everything is fine.* Only that is an illusion. We cannot in truth know that, save for that exact moment, everything is fine. As it is said, life can change on a dime. The illusion of certainty, that *Whew, everything is fine*, comes at a cost to the phobic person of the anxiety of the phobia. Another way to say this is that in order for a person not to suffer phobic anxiety, he or she will have to face and deal with the ongoing uncertainties of life.

When I listen to Laing and to Semrad, I take it that my task as a therapist is to accompany my patients, to help them to identify and bear the pain of life they cannot bear alone. If I form an image to represent this process, I see patient and therapist bobbing along in an ocean of existential pain, the patient rendered more buoyant and comforted by their connection. As I get on with the work, I find myself increasingly drawn to the writings of the British pediatrician-become-psychiatrist Donald W. Winnicott, who emphasizes the creative potential of the connection between the patient and the therapist. When I read Winnicott's writings, the image I have is of patient and therapist playing in the sand at the ocean shore, sometimes tunneling toward each other, sometimes working busily side by side, and sometimes rocking back on their heels to look at what they are making and at what they have made.

Twenty years after I first hear R. D. Laing, it happens that he comes again to speak in Boston, this time sponsored by Interface, a New Age organization. As before, the crowd desiring attendance cannot be accommodated in the usual space. This time the talk is moved to a high school auditorium. Laing is still much as I remember him—handsome, charismatic, and with a brogue. His speech is entitled "On Myths of Love," about themes in Greek mythology that bear on the challenge of loving commitment to another while trying to be true to oneself.

Fortunate to be among the few to have the opportunity to ask a question at the completion of Laing's remarks, I put this to him:

> *Twenty years ago you said that the work of a therapist was to help our patients to tolerate uncertainty. Would you say the same thing now?*

Laing's reply:

> *I remember that. Yes. I would say that. But I would also say that the work is to help the patient to be in the presence of the*

other [*someone other than him- or herself*], *and that* that *requires tolerating a great deal of uncertainty!*

It appears that Laing has evolved from helping keep patients afloat in the ocean of existential pain to working with the interplay of *self* and *other-than-self*, which has been my own evolution as a therapist as well.

Fundamental to this work, and unchanging in its application and value, is what I learned from Semrad about the importance of sadness and grief in coming to terms with life. In Semrad's words:

Sorrow is the vitamin of growth.

Wanting something to *be* when it *is not*—or wanting something *to be other than it is*—is a standard of the human condition. A familiar response to such frustration is anger—anger that represents a holding on to the wished-for element. Semrad taught that getting on with life requires surrendering to the sadness that accompanies letting go of the wished-for element. With time, the natural process of grief eases, and the energy formerly tied up with the wished-for element becomes freed up to attach to something or someone that is available. We have to let go of what's not available anymore so that we can attach to what *is*.

This is what we residents learned those years in the 1960s while pop-psych philosophies proliferated, encouraging patients to "get the anger out" by shouting and beating mattresses with battaccas (padded bats). Certainly, anger is a useful indicator of what matters to a person. But identifying and connecting with anger alone will keep a person stalled in a cycle of rage and self-pity. Growth can happen only through surrendering to sadness.

Semrad's teaching was brilliant, as well, at focusing on a person's responsibility for him- or herself. Sympathetic but steady, he would investigate the part we play in what happens to us. In my work with patients, in an appropriate context, I find it valuable to make use of his words. With the disarming acknowledgment that this question can be challenged, I can offer: "As my teacher, Dr. Semrad used to say, 'How did you make him do that to you?'" I am one step removed from holding the person responsible for his or her circumstance, which allows both of us to look at the matter in a usefully inquiring way.

An old medical school aphorism—*see one, do one, teach one*—applied in its way to residency training. As first-year residents, we began supervising medical students. As third-year residents, we supervised first-year residents. When I completed all three years of training, I began private practice of psychiatry and also accepted a Harvard teaching appointment on the staff at Mass Mental, where, for the next seven years, I provided supervision to residents for several hours each week.

For me, a high point of teaching here was the opportunity to have some ongoing contact with Dr. Semrad. From time to time, he would refer a private patient to me, which occasioned another meeting point—and a couple of times a year, I'd knock on his office door for a casual chat. In September 1976, after

Semrad's August vacation break, I stopped in to see him. A few weeks later, on October 7, 1976, at midday I was at Mass Mental wrapping up a couple of hours of supervision. My schedule was such that I had to hop in my car immediately to make it back for an appointment with a patient in my private office. That day I dawdled in the administration office for half an hour, considering the pros and cons of going up to knock on Semrad's door. Reluctantly I decided against importuning him for nothing in particular. Unaccountably, I simply did not want to leave the hospital. Finally, more than half an hour late, I raced to my car and back to my office.

Later that afternoon, a colleague phoned with jolting news. Dr. Semrad had died. A heart attack in his sleep while he napped on his analytic couch after lunch . . . *while I was hanging on at Mass Mental, having a hard time getting myself to leave.*

I miss him still.

Twelve

Second Marriage

My *second marriage was a mess. Not that we didn't* know what we were in for. Several times in several years we had tried to let go of each other, but there was no help for it— the only way out led straight through marriage to divorce.

B. was often funny. One of his more graceless jokes was his occasional habit of introducing me as his "first wife." Our romantic connection of sexual passion and intellectual excitement lacked compassionate heart. It allowed an illusion of intimacy, but suffered without the ballast of emotional maturity. Each of us had a way to go to clarity about and acceptance of inside and outside realities. Semrad used to say (and surely the meaning transcends the grammar): "Everyone has to buy peace between their head, their heart, and their body." For sure I felt alive with B., but peace for us? No way.

Why couldn't it work? For one thing, he was a man unable to make a commitment to a pair of shoes. He would shop to find just the right ones—take a good long time about it, then make the purchase. Most often, he'd bring them back the next day. He had decided that they were somehow not quite right.

I remember the Georg Kepec painting with the sandy-textured paint that hung for more than a year above the fire-place. I got to like it quite a lot. The gallery owner thought that it was sold, although some money was owed; but after a year, back it was in the gallery. It wasn't a matter of the money.

B. had just as tough a time settling on a career path. If I remember the details correctly, he had made it into law school and quit the first week. He had begun studies to become a rabbi, and then left. He had completed most of the work toward a master's degree in religion and philosophy, and then dropped out. At the time I met him, in 1968, he was working in a computer company and considering applying to medical school. He was in therapy and was himself interested in becoming a psychiatrist. Only after our divorce did I learn that he had been applying to medical schools in Europe and having the mailings sent to his parents' home, so that I wouldn't know about his potential plans.

While B. certainly touched me physically and was intellectually engageable, in other ways he was as unreachable as my mother had been and as out of touch with me emotionally. Semrad's observation: "The hope of the repetition compulsion: that next time will be better!"

Unquestionably I had married men with whom I repeated the experience of unfulfilled longing for connection and closeness that had been a significant aspect of my relationship with my mother, and I know I had had the hope to "make it better" each time. To have broken the pattern, I would have had to deal with the source—to see my mother more clearly, to recognize my experience with her for what it had been, to feel the anger and the sadness that went with it, to accept the reality that it could never be "fixed," and to grieve until I had made my peace. When I was thirty and chose to marry B., I was not yet there.

He and I were, at the time, each so much concerned with our individual struggles with life that we had little loving support for one another. I don't know which was worse: his acknowledged lack of capacity for empathy, which he accepted as a quirk of character, or my belief that I *was* empathic, oblivious to the limits of my ability, at times, to get beyond myself.

Each of us was so much attached to developing and holding on to our individual living arrangements that, even after we married, we did not take on the challenge of creating a home together. For most of the time, although he lived with me, he kept his apartment. I found the idea of this disturbing but the actuality of it really quite fine—since I didn't want to accommodate much of his furniture or many of his *things* in what I continued to feel was *my* home.

We terrified each other. He needed his space, or so it

seemed; I needed reassurance of connection, it appeared. What I came to understand, much later, was that his was the fear of abandonment, and mine the need *not* to be crowded. Ingenious, the way we managed to take care of ourselves—he by distancing at the reassurance of connection, guaranteeing my pursuit and his ongoing experience of being wanted; I by pursuing until the reassurance of temporary connection, never being threatened by engulfment, since he dependably pulled back. We were both terrified of intimacy.

We married in 1970. Our wedding reception took place, fittingly, on a magnificent but permanently moored ship, the S.S. *Peter Stuyvesant* at Anthony's Pier 4 restaurant in Boston. Trying to get the marriage afloat and moving occupied the better part of five years, during which I learned more of what I importantly needed to learn about being alone than what I needed equally to learn about intimacy. Painfully, it was as hard for us to let go of each other as it was to be partners. After the 1975 divorce, we vacationed one more time together, leasing a house in Jamaica next door to Eddie Fisher's villa, Borborygmus (the medical term for "stomach growling"!), with cases of empty Dom Pérignon bottles in the courtyard. Eventually my prayers not to want him were answered, and the connection faded into history.

Several years later, while happily stranded on vacation in Puerto Rico by airport closings due to the blizzard of '78, reading newspaper stories reporting on the storm in the northeastern United States, I saw an Associated Press wire photo showing the S. S. *Peter Stuyvesant* in Boston Harbor. Damaged by the pounding it had taken on its moorings next to

Anthony's restaurant, it was listing, half-sunk and sinking in the storm. *The marriage couldn't make it, but did the ship have to go down, too?* I thought also that if the *Peter Stuyvesant* had been whole and seaworthy, free of its tether, it might well have made it through afloat.

I cannot measure the proportions of chance and choice that bear on my untethered life. I do know that "whole and seaworthy" is an apt caption of the qualities I trust and value in a human being.

Thirteen

Mothering

I've always rankled against what I consider to be the stupidity of misguided egocentric application of the so-called Golden Rule. What if the person you are "doing unto" does not appreciate, or even want, something as you would have done unto you? Opportunities for attending to this distinction certainly presented themselves in my relationship with my daughter. From the earliest days, Jenni demonstrated a personality quite different from mine. As a child, I had longed for attention of an inquiring kind. My little girl pretty regularly rebuffed my natural attentiveness and interest in her experience. Jennifer treasured privacy and was most comfortable keeping her own counsel. In the face of what I suffered in not being seen clearly and treated respectfully in my childhood, I wished particularly to support my daughter's autonomy and to nourish her sense of self. When she was only about seven I had occasion to think that perhaps I had done too good a job.

It happened in an instant, in the foyer of the dining room of Boston's Ritz-Carlton Hotel. I was there, waiting for Jennifer and B., my second husband, to arrive. Some mix-up had occurred. We were supposed to have met up someplace else earlier but had somehow missed the connection. I figured that surely they would join me at the Ritz, where a reservation for dinner had definitely been made.

After what seemed like a very long time, the two of them finally turned up. Jennifer looked up at B., who had apparently insisted on waiting for me elsewhere, and said, "I told you she'd probably be here." But to me, Jenni said, "Mom, I didn't think I was ever going to see you again, and I didn't have a chance to say good-bye."

Oh my god. Seven years old and she could *imagine* saying good-bye to me—and going on without me. I had a confusion of feelings: pain and regret at the anxiety she had suffered in the mix-up, an odd sense of accomplishment at having raised a child with the capacity at age seven to conceive of herself as a separate being who could imagine grieving the loss of her mother, and hurt at having been so readily dispensed with, if only in her imagination.

What glimpses I was allowed into Jenni's inner life were precious to me. Even today, the yellowing pages in a folder of her sixth-grade writings—a school assignment to describe life on an imaginary planet—are the first things I would save from a fire. Jennifer's creation was a place she named Callo, inhabited by Callowins. A couple of excerpts of the most innocently touching parts (punctuation and spelling intact):

Callowins have no clocks; they have a built-in time mechanism. All people are vegetarians.

BIRTH

Everytime a woman is pregnant and is ready for deliverance she goes to section four and forgets about time. She just delivers her baby. (with the help of her husband) When the baby is born, they change the population and make it one more. She forgets about time to take care of her baby and teach the baby how to plant.

Here is their scedule: . . . 7:00pm to 8:00 go to section four and mourn for the dead or rejoice the new born.

When I read Jenni's references to "forgetting about time," I could not but understand these as expressions of her wish that she and I could live without a schedule, and that we could spend much more time together. This made me sad for both of us. I could take comfort, though, that my daughter was so clearly in touch with and creatively expressive of this wish, and I was awed by her poignant awareness of the realities of death and of life, of mourning the dead and rejoicing the newborn, of mothers, and husbands, and babies. I was re-assured that she seemed to be getting enough of what she needed to become a whole, alive person. I liked to think that I had given her much of what mattered.

Another challenge, as well as gift, for Jennifer was her physical beauty, an endowment that from childhood she accepted without vanity, later used to advantage in an acting career, and has mostly enjoyed. Today it knocks me out when anyone notes a resemblance between us. Save for the high-cheekboned Russian elements and some resonance of soul coming through the eyes, I think we do not look alike. I'm fine with this, as I am with most of the differences between us. The one difference I rued was Jenni's lack of interest in reading the books I had saved from my childhood, not just the picture books of my earliest years, whose illustrations I could almost *taste*, but also the substantial ones.

I still have the copy of my absolute favorite, *Little Women*, a book I read so many times that I can quote passages from memory. In particular, I identified with Jo, the writer with glorious long tresses. I was in awe of Jo's sacrifice in selling her hair to help her family at a time of crisis. When I first read the book, I had finally been allowed to let my Dutch clip grow out, and I couldn't imagine choosing to part with my ponytail. For most of my life, actually, I have worn my hair long. When, as sometimes happens, someone remarks on the mane with which I am blessed, Marmee's comment to Jo springs into my mind: *O Jo . . . Your one beauty . . .*

My confidently beautiful daughter always loved being read

to and loved picture books, but when eventually it came to reading on her own, she opted, mostly, not to. In 1969, when she was in first grade, dyslexia wasn't understood as it is today. In second grade, a "reading teacher" gave extra attention to some of the children, and while Jenni did learn to read, it was apparent that she didn't enjoy it. In retrospect, I am sure that her lack of pleasure in reading was a consequence of some dyslexic process.

Passion for acting—and fundamental intelligence—carried Jennifer through college. On graduating, she came up with an efficient way to support herself while trying to make it as an actress in New York: Jenni became proficient at a word-processing software program designed for use by law firms. She also began to tutor other acting-hopefuls in this skill, which offered the prospect of more reliable and better income than did waiting tables. For Jennifer, the computer work produced an additional benefit. Typing complex material sometimes from recorded dictation, sometimes from handwritten revision to existing documents, and sometimes from her own revisions resulted, ultimately, in Jenni's becoming an excellent writer and an extraordinarily fine editor. I speculate that her work at the computer promoted some neurological patterning that counterbalanced whatever dyslexic process may have been in play.

Jenni did meet with a decent measure of success as an actor, but after seven years, she made a decision I would never have imagined. At the culmination of months of private distress, Jennifer telephoned in some anguish to tell me that she was tired of "spending more time looking for [acting] work than working" and that she was seriously considering giving it up. Acting had been her passion since she was six, and I was sympathetic but otherwise quiet at the news.

Following the phone call, my attention was not extraordinarily focused on my daughter's dilemma—something I didn't realize at the time to be milestone evidence that she and I had achieved some considerable degree of wholesome separateness. My own early experience of having been pressed with interfering advice when I was faced with important life decisions, together with my trust in Jenni's ability to choose her own path, figured large in this as well. I can say, truly, that I was surprised at Jennifer's subsequent announcement. She had, indeed, decided to give up her career in theatre—to become a lawyer.

Gellebbed yorren, my mother would have said. The two-word Yiddish phrase translates to: "Imagine living to see this wonderful and satisfying development"—the experience of watching Jenni blossom in law school. I did greatly enjoy witnessing Jennifer's pleasure in the work when, in her second year, she was chosen to teach legal writing to first-year students. These days, *gellebbed yorren* to its ultimate: I am appreciative when Jennifer finds the time to look over a manuscript for me. I value particularly her ability to come up with the subtle adjustments that improve for clarity and grace the words and structure of a piece, tampering least with the original writing.

Last year, juggling the demands of work and family, Jennifer put me on notice not to expect her to read through my new book before I sent it to the publisher. When the due date approached, I took a couple of weeks away from psychiatric practice and installed myself, laptop, research files, printer, and all, in a rented house in Chatham, by the sea, to work full-time on the manuscript. In mid-May, when I finished, I was rewarded with a weekend visit to Jenni and her family and the festivity of our annual Mother's Day brunch. I leveraged the occasion to ask my daughter, albeit hesitantly, whether she might, in the next couple of days, give a quick read to my manuscript. Jenni evaded the request. I'm afraid that she is good at that sort of thing, too.

When we got to dessert, apologizing for not having had time to shop for a gift, my daughter presented me with the card she had written earlier:

> *This entitles the bearer to one editorial read-through*
> *of the completed manuscript.*

This was the occasion upon which my granddaughter learned that sometimes people cry when they are happy. With a full heart, I wrote, in the Acknowledgments of my last book: *"Dearest Jenni, you nourished my spirit when I needed it most. No author could have a more exquisitely discerning, critical, respectful, balanced, and intelligent reader."*

As fate has it, Jennifer's daughter, Alexandra, was born with a brain very much like my own. By the time she was eighteen months old, Alexandra had made friends with the letters—all except the *F*, that is. A magnetic alphabet went up on the refrigerator, and Alexandra at eighteen months said, *Mommy, take away the F. Don't yike the F.*

Whatever it was about the *F* that required its banishment

remained a mystery, but another of Alexandra's unique requests did eventuate in an explanation. The year of the *F* was the year of Tiger Woods's record-setting fifteen-stroke-margin win at the U.S. Open at Pebble Beach. Camera-panned drives following an indiscernible golf ball through the air are not my idea of compelling television viewing, but Tiger Woods at Pebble Beach was a happening. It began to seem as though Woods could hit a golf ball from California to Boston in four strokes. Alexandra, age two, was visiting me at the time, and I pointed him out to her on the television screen: "That's Tiger Woods. He hits the ball in the hole."

Three years later, when she was five, Alexandra and I had our first experience hitting the ball in the hole—miniature golf at a nifty little course complete with traps, both sand and water, in Orleans on Cape Cod. A few months later, when we set out to play again, Alexandra asked, please, if we could play at some other course. This request was easy enough to accommodate, and we enjoyed a couple of rounds at a simple little course in Harwichport. When I ventured to ask why she hadn't wanted to play at Orleans:

ALEX: I don't like it when my ball goes into the water.
  ME: Ohhhhhhh . . . you know, I don't think that Tiger
          Woods likes it when his ball goes in the water, either.
ALEX: You mean he plays at *that* place?

This delightful little girl may eventually enjoy reading some of the books I've been saving for fifty-five years. I am not sure how the sensibility of a child of the twenty-first century will take to the likes of the Bobbsey Twins, the Five Little Peppers, and the Nancy Drew mysteries, some of whose once-compelling features are now at best, quaint. The timeless elements and classic writing of *Little Women*, *Understood Betsy*, and *The Secret Garden* more dependably await. At five, Alexandra has it planned that she will, herself, have four children: "two girls and two boys." Come to think of it, maybe she *will* like the Bobbsey Twins . . .

Fourteen

Finding My Father

A_t *the cusp of 1982–83 I am spending Christmas and* New Year's in Mexico with my sophomore-in-college daughter, both of us visiting Yvette, a former housekeeper who has become a friend. Yvette is a Frenchwoman who lived with us when Jenni was eight and nine, and who, for a time, I suspected of being an international spy. This idea was more a function of her capacity for privacy together with mine for paranoia than of any evidence of substance. The fact that when she left our household Yvette moved to China did fuel my fantasy, though. Her subsequent move has been to Mexico, where, in 1982, she lives with her sweetheart, Miguel, on the outskirts of Acapulco.

The second week in January 1983: Jenni and I have enjoyed our time with Yvette and Miguel and have had a warm and adventuresome time together in the countryside at Pié de la Cuesta, where only the bedrooms and kitchen alcove of our rented rustic villa on the blue Pacific are fully protected from the elements, and where, in this year of the first major devaluation of the peso, I'm not so sure that we are adequately protected from the banditos whose gunshots we hear in the distance, sometimes, in the night. Thankfully our safety has not been threatened. We have had one particularly memorable daytime adventure, though.

The day we arrived, we noticed a roadside billboard that invited a visit to PLAYA SAN JERÓNIMO, a beach FABULOSO, and only 26 KILÓMETROS distant. This is comfortably within range for a day's excursion, we think, when we set out in our rented car, expecting a short drive and a lazy day in the sun. The first hitch happens several miles down the road: we meet up with a roadblock and Mexican police. They look us over, check out the car, open the trunk, and finally wave us ahead. Jenni decides that they are looking for drugs. Whatever they are up to, I am glad they let this *gringa* and her daughter move on.

Drive on we do. And on and on. Here comes a billboard: PLAYA SAN JERÓNIMO, 26 KILÓMETROS. Huh? I estimate that we've driven about twenty kilometers already, but continue hopefully for another stretch. Up comes another billboard: PLAYA SAN JERÓNIMO, 30 KILÓMETROS. Stymied, when we drive through what looks to be a town, we stop to ask. My Spanish is really pretty decent, and the blank stares and shrugs I get when I mention Playa San Jerónimo draw the comment from Jenni that maybe we have come upon a town where the population has intermarried to the detriment of their cognitive faculties. In the growing heat of midmorning, we begin to feel as though we have entered a Mexican twilight zone. Not ready to quit, we drive a bit farther, and here comes another billboard with the clincher: GRACIAS POR VISITAR PLAYA SAN JERÓNIMO (*Thank you for visiting San Jerónimo Beach*).

I figure that Mexican tourism promoters probably put up signs first and get around to developing the site mañana. I think that maybe they had an oversupply of the 26 KILÓMETROS signs and didn't want them to go to waste. We shrug and turn around for home. At one point, our road winds along above and parallel to a river where, at midday, women are scrubbing laundry on rocks at the shoreline—white sheets spread on boulders to dry. Goats graze near the roadside, where the most primitive of open-air restaurants offers the possibility of lunch.

Caution to the winds—*We've got to make something of this outing*—we stop to eat and are served a kind of stew ladled from a bubbling pot and tortillas slapped together while we watch, cooked on a hot flat rock over a wood fire. The food tastes delicious. "Chicken and beans, this is chicken and beans," I tell Jenni and myself, hopefully. I don't want to look at the goats. Flies are buzzing around the food, but I think *everything is hot, hot, hot—no germs will have survived*. At least in the matter of ingesting the meal without later incident, my intention prevails, but we never, ever forget our day at Playa San Jerónimo.

Jenni's winter vacation comes to its end. When she leaves to return to Penn State I stay on, awaiting the arrival of my father, whom I've invited to join me in Mexico. This time last year we were skidding into the extended nightmare of my mother's terminal illness: six months of kidney failure, dialysis, and congestive heart failure—an all-around brutal time.

This is a new year, and for my dad to vacation with me is new ground.

Pleasure and relaxation were not hallmarks of the life of my family of origin. The sad truth is that even in my adulthood, my mother and I never managed to find a comfortable way to be together. I couldn't get myself to give up trying, though. During one of our last times together, when I noticed that her skin was very dry, I picked up the lotion bottle. She did allow me to apply it, but when I began to massage her gently, my mother pulled away abruptly. "It's too greasy" was what she said. I had every reason to have known the futility of it, but I was still hoping for some connection of loving touch with my mother.

Some events of the last year were a true horror. One evening, I answered my home telephone to hear my mother, calling from her bed in a Worcester hospital, gasping desperately for breath. I knew enough about the parameters of her medical condition to recognize that she was in congestive heart failure. Her lungs were flooded with fluids and she was actually drowning. Urgently I got through to the nursing station to report the emergency, and then raced the forty miles to the hospital. I arrived to find the attending physician performing kidney dialysis to remove the excess fluid. Thankfully, my mother had begun to breathe easier. The near catastrophe had been the result of an I.V. running fully open, even though her kidneys were not functioning. Her body had not been able to handle the fluid load.

My mother managed to survive this perilously close call, but she didn't have the physical margin to hold on much longer. The next crisis was to be her last. After her death, relief, unease about the relief, and sadness for the unhappiness of her life jockeyed for primacy. It has taken decades for the intensity of these feelings to fade.

While she lived, my mother compelled family attention. She was a hub that kept my dad and me focused on her and at the same time at some distance from one another. Once she was no longer with us, I found myself hoping that he and I might find a way to connect and to enjoy something of life. In particular, I wanted to come to some ease with him. I wished for something more grounded and sustainable than the excitement I had felt for him in my early childhood, a life of feelings of which no living spark remains.

Zorba's colorful metaphor for life—"the full catastrophe"—is the way I've always thought about the particular tangle of what is familiarly known as Oedipal stuff. The dynamics are universal, the details tedious, and the consequences costly when a developing child cannot manage well enough, for whatever reasons particular to his or her family, to relinquish longings to win the exclusive love of one or the other parent, leave them to each other, and eventually go off to find a primary connection of his or her own.

Although of personal psychotherapy I had plenty, it was not in psychotherapy that I gained a workable understanding of these human struggles. That happened in my experience with my mentor, Dr. Semrad.

On point here—two simple truths in his plain words:

The only way a father and daughter can part is to acknowledge how much they love one another. As long as they "hate" each other, they stick together like glue.

Every time you put a mile between a father and a daughter, her heart aches a little.

I remember the feelings of my little-girlhood—the excitement of waiting for my dad to come home from work, bringing his energy, smell, and feel into the house. One sharp and early memory: standing at sink level while he shaved. I almost couldn't watch. It was okay when he lathered the brush in the Old Spice mug and rubbed it in circles on his face and throat. But then he fitted a razor blade into its holder, leaned up close to the bathroom mirror, and, pulling the skin tight to meet it, scraped the edge over his face. Sometimes, when he swiped the razor over his soaped throat, a red tinge came up—a bit of blood he stanched with a stinging white styptic pencil. He taught me these words: *stanched* and *styptic*.

My dad was strong, lithe, and, to me, handsome. With age,

he came to look a lot like Art Carney, but when he was younger his features were more refined, and he resembled Robert Stack. In contrast to that actor's style of quiet self-assurance, however, my dad's was a boyish bravado. Balancing with his palms on the floor, he would demonstrate that he could stand on his head. Like a circus performer, in his grocery store he would swing in circles a large paper sack of potatoes clenched in his teeth. With a child's conviction, I remember thinking, *My dad can do anything.* He was, actually, very clever, and he taught me, early, to solve problems outside the envelope. So caught up was I in pride at my dad's ingenuity, I never considered appalling an aphorism he chanted like a moral dictum: *There's more than one way to skin a cat.*

One particular image endures from the summer of 1943, when my mother and I, in the company of my grandmother, Auntie Rosie, Uncle Bob, and their kids, went for a week's vacation to Revere Beach, on the north shore of Boston, where we stayed in a rooming house of some kind. I remember Auntie Rosie's delicious homemade potato chips, which she cooked in the shared common kitchen. I don't remember how we made the trip from Worcester, but my dad came with us just for the weekend, and then had to return home to go to work.

The memory of seeing him off at the bus stop still gives me an ache at the bottom of my throat. It was wartime. Soldiers and sailors in uniform were everywhere. I knew that my dad was simply going home, but as I watched him climb up the steps to get on the bus alone, the worry and sadness I felt were such that he might as well have been leaving to fight overseas. *Every time you put a mile between a father and a daughter, her heart aches a little.* Within two years, and by the time I was five, my dad came to own the ~~grocery~~ store that came to own him. He worked dawn to dark, and our special times together were no more.

Four decades later, January 1983 in Mexico, hoping for a new beginning, I am waiting for my dad at the Acapulco airport. This extraordinary vacation is a challenge from the moment he steps off the plane. *Ohmygod, he has colored his hair, can it be, orange? Oh hell, he looks like a clown.* I don't want to admit to myself that more than ever I wish he were like my uncle Al— solid, sure of himself, easily attentive, classy, and bald. Fat chance. I have to remind myself not to give in to what I usually do when I'm with my parents: go on automatic or withdraw. *Okay, just be yourself and stay right here, right with him.*

The easy part is the gladness I feel when he is happy. I've always appreciated my dad's zest for life. At sixty-eight, his experience of travel, a handful of occasions in all, has been up and down the East Coast, Maine to Miami. But his imagination has taken him on great adventures. He dreams of flamenco dancing and bullfighting in Spain, *the great Bob Mandell* a featured performer. I have heard that Dad did win some ballroom-dancing contests in Springfield in the 1930s. I have no trouble imagining him as a torero with cape and sword. *My dad can do anything.*

Anything, that is, with the exception of seeing or hearing what's going on for someone else. To be sure, he sees and hears *something.* Whenever I start to try to tell him anything, he interrupts with a response linked either to his first association or to his idea of where my comment may be going. This time, I am determined to hang in there. "Dad, you're not *listening* to me." "Dad, you don't even know what I was trying to say." "Dad, please let me finish." And, pretty loud: "Dad, please *listen* to me." I have never tried so hard. I even explain to him when I shout that I am shouting because I want to have a better relationship with him. *I want to be there.*

He loves it.

In response to my noise, he doesn't raise his voice. He never gets angry. He simply says, "I'm glad that our relationship is important to you" and goes right on being *the great Bob Mandell.*

When I'm not trying to talk to him we do have some good times. He loves the *quebrada,* where the young men dive off the cliff into the sea. We watch a lot of divers timing their leap for the critical depth of the incoming waves. *He could have done it when he was younger.* We watch the sunset from Club Náutico, at Pié de la Cuesta—to which with fractured Spanish and gusto he will refer for years to come. Familiarly, I see the world through his eyes. I know his experience and join in some of it with pleasure. *I wish he could see me, know me.* I keep trying. *Dad, please listen to me.* After three days, I am exhausted, disheartened at the failure of connection with my father. I'm ready to return home tomorrow, as planned, relieved by Yvette, who will oversee the remainder of my father's stay.

Finally, it is our last day. The recent devaluation of the peso has been a windfall for purchases made with American currency, and it's hard to believe what a dollar can buy. My dad has bought a pair of leather "goucho" (as he calls them) boots and wants to shop some more. More than ready for a break, I suggest that we separate and meet up after a while. I'll check out the other side of the Costera, the many-lane divided highway that runs past the strip of resort hotels and shops where street vendors hawk and barter on the sidewalks, their shouts barely audible above the cacophony of the traffic. With no signal lights, the Costera is hazardous.

I make it across, busy myself with something or other, and then it's time to meet up again. I've made it halfway back, to the grassy median, when I catch sight of my dad walking away on the far sidewalk. Even though I realize that my voice will not carry above the din, I have the urge to call to him to stop and wait for me. I try anyway. *"D-a-a-a-a-d! D-a-a-a-a-d!"* I can barely hear myself. He stops and looks around, head jerking and eyes darting. *"D-a-a-a-a-d!"* Like a bird who hears its young potentially in danger and can discern its chirping from the noise of the surround, my father hears me.

I know the grounding of another aspect of the archetypal connection. This deep knowing stays. Something in me relaxes for the first time.

Fifteen

Natural Passage

September 1988. My daughter has been engaged to be married for the past festive and rainy year. Jennifer has always loved parties and celebrations. She loves planning them, making lists. Jenni loves making lists more than anything. As a child, she even made lists to keep track of the coming year's school grade assignments and the social pairings of her thirty-one dolls, who lived an active life in a room upstairs under the eaves. Jennifer did this each fall, until she was a sophomore in college and we carefully put the dolls away.

Amid the clutter in her bedroom and crumpled in her

wastebasket, the lists are like diary pages. Privacy to be respected.

Happily busy with many lists this past year, Jenni has had much to think about and to arrange, beginning with the engagement party and leading up to the wedding, the wedding, the wedding. Weddings are the best for lists, she says. In fact, as the wedding day grows near and the list-making days dwindle to few, she brightly comments that she could be happy with a career as a wedding planner.

Careful planning saved the day for last year's engagement party, for sure, scheduled for September in our Boston suburb. Talking to the tent person, we consider our chances for a warm, dry day. We order side panels and heaters, and it's a good thing. The day of the party, as my mother (may her soul rest in peace) would have said, it rains cats and dogs. Even in her gossamer frock, Jenni glows, warmed both with excitement and by the tent heaters. Those of us a little less excited are grateful for the heaters.

Since the kickoff of the engagement party, each wedding-related occasion has been blessed with rain, and not merely a sprinkle. The shower guests carried real umbrellas. The brides-maids' luncheon required boots as well. The wedding will happen in mid-September at a North Shore castle. Built by an English actor in the 1920s, Stillington Hall is set amid beautiful formal gardens overlooking the sea. *A perfect place for an outdoor ceremony and cocktail reception before the dinner*, we dare to dream. But we are New Englanders and know better than to count on the weather. Remembering that the castle has stone fireplaces and candle-laden sconces, we are comforted with romantic images of warmth and light. Sunshine and champagne in the gardens overlooking the sea would be lovely, though.

The week before the wedding, I begin to feel something of a different level of consciousness—an experience I have had at times of major life transitions in the past. My internal atmosphere is ionized with something. I find myself making a kind of shrine on the dining room table of photographs of the women in my family who cannot be with us at the wedding: my mother, my grandmother, Auntie Rosie, Auntie Bess. I have some discomfort when I think "shrine." Jews are not supposed to make shrines—graven images and all that. But mostly I am comforted every time I walk past the dining room and look in.

My masseuse is a Buddhist with a real shrine. Actually, she has two—one in her kitchen and one in her bedroom. The kitchen one gets cornmeal; the bedroom one gets incense. On the massage table, I tell her that I am thinking it would be nice if we could have a warm day with some sunshine for the wedding. She suggests that I get some cornmeal, go into my backyard, and throw it into each of the four directions, asking of the winds that my wish be granted "if it be for the good of all."

The week before the wedding, twice each day I perform the ritual. With a sack of cornmeal from the natural-food store, I go into the backyard. Feeling pagan, I dare to stand and move in a circle, facing east, south, west, and then north, throwing handfuls of cornmeal into the air and speaking aloud to the winds. "Please, if it be for the good of all the universe, let it be fair on Sunday."

The day before the wedding, the forecast predicts rain.

My daughter and I are sitting at the kitchen table when she glances into the backyard and says, "Mom, come here and take a look. There are a whole bunch of robins out there. I've never seen so many robins before."

Before I understand my reaction, I feel goose bumps rise on my arms and legs. Consciousness comes slowly. *Robin redbreast* was a feature of my mother's language. I have never, ever seen so many robins.

And then I know. Of course—the cornmeal. The robins have come to eat the cornmeal. The pictures on the dining room table and the cornmeal have brought to this archetypal rite of passage the spirits of my mother, my aunts, my grandmother. They come with me and warm me the following day, as the monsoons pour down, blessing my daughter's wedding. Blessing her marriage.

Sixteen

True Reflection

Sublimation, *I learned in high school chemistry class, is* the technical term for the process through which solid matter converts directly into gas. The use of the term in psychology to mean *a defense mechanism through which the individual satisfies one instinctive drive through the substitution of another behavior* is a bit of a puzzle. Maybe what's meant is that a solid instinctive drive—*I want to clobber my boss*—can be vaporized and dispersed by substitute behavior: *Go, Jets, Go!* I don't much use the lingo of psychology, and I do appreciate the metaphoric elegance of some scientific descriptives—all this a somewhat cumbersome explanation of my use of one word in the following sentence . . .

One spring day when I am nearly sixty, the stubborn self-criticism that has not yielded to decades of inner work sublimates and evaporates in the noonday sun, catalyzed by an expression on the innocent face of my one-year-old granddaughter.

It happens in the park on the grounds of Wellesley City Hall. My friend Jeanne, who lives in that town and has been a particular favorite of Alexandra's since the day they met, comes with us to visit the ducks. Alexandra toddles happily up and down a little bridge over a brook, stares at the other babies, delights in the ducks, and begins to explore the rest of the scene. Enormous old trees, newly leafed, offer shade, and a few wooden picnic tables the hospitality of a place to sit for refreshment.

Keeping an eye on her unsteady toddling, I notice Alexandra beginning to draw back. Following her sidelong gaze, I see that she is fixed on a picnic table upon which, full length, fully clothed, and supine, lies a large man. The image is a strange one, and Alexandra is clearly frightened. Quickly I say: "It's okay, sweetheart. It's just a man taking a nap in the sun. He looks funny, doesn't he, lying on the table like that? Everything is all right. He's just taking a nap in the sun." She has had enough of the park for this day, and we head for home.

An epiphany for me: the look in the eyes I saw on Alexandra's face is a mirror of my child-self. For me, though, no single event accounted for an underlying and continuing experience of puzzlement and fear. Vigilance and dread were not passing miseries; and, worse for me, nobody noticed.

I began to understand the roots of these troubles early in my psychiatric training, in the late 1960s, when I discovered Winnicott's writings that addressed the crucial matter of "self and other-than-self" in ways at the same time practical and poetic. The titles of a couple of Winnicott's books—*The Child, the Family, and the Outside World* and (my favorite) *Playing and Reality*—give an idea of his range of focus.

Dr. Donald W. Winnicott was a brilliantly creative psychoanalyst and specialist in childhood emotional development. I was drawn in particular to his conception and lucid description of the critically important role of the parent or caretaker of a baby in reflecting back accurately that which the baby is experiencing. For the most part this occurs naturally in the course of living, often nonverbally and sometimes with words. The key matter is that the baby's experience be seen clearly, so that the reflection is a true one. Winnicott made the point that being responded to on the basis of being seen clearly both helps a baby learn to know her- or himself and establishes a foundation for trust in the outside world.

My training in child psychiatry left me with the sense that whatever I can do to help parents better care for a child is oftentimes more effective than whatever I may be able to accomplish directly with a small child in my office. It is the parents, after all, who create and sustain the child's environment and who respond to the child's steady needs. Occasionally I find it useful to meet together with a mother and her baby or toddler, in order to observe the interaction between them.

One particular experience in my private practice of psychiatry demonstrates how a simple acknowledgment of one child's experience helped her to manage strong feelings. In this instance, I am working with a young mother who has consulted me for help with some difficulties of her own. One day she tells me that she is at her wits' end with the angry outbursts of her three-year-old daughter, whose tantrums have escalated since the birth of a baby brother. I decide to meet, once, with the little girl.

Lilly, at three, is pretty sharp. I get out a large pad of paper and some crayons to play "the squiggle game," a game devised by Winnicott. First I scribble a large abstract scrawl on the paper, then invite Lilly to "make it into something." Next it is Lilly's turn to scribble a scrawl, and my turn to "make it into something." Lilly isn't particularly interested in playing the squiggle game by my rules. Instead, she takes the black crayon and begins to print, large, saying; "I can make a *W*; I can make a *W*."

W W

Below the *W*'s, she goes on drawing: "I can make an M; I can make an M."

W W
M M

I look at what she has drawn, take another crayon, and make a couple of circles:

o   o

W W
M M

I say: "Wow, Look at what you have made—a face with big teeth!"

Lilly gets up and begins running and dancing around the room, and soon the session is over. We say good-bye.

The following week, her mother begins by asking what in the world I could have done that has settled Lilly down. Apparently the little girl has been relaxed and pretty happy since our meeting. I take out the drawing with the M's and W's, and both of us are impressed with the relief Lilly experienced simply by having her feelings seen, accepted, and reflected back to her accurately.

That incredible day in the park with Alexandra and the man on the picnic table brought me face to face with the realization that, as a child, I had been as innocent and as good as she. My friend Jeanne's witness to this event in the context of all that she knows of me helped bring the realization of my childhood innocence home for good.

A few months later, another sunny day in another park with Alexandra occasions joy of equivalent healing power.

Alexandra is sixteen months old that August afternoon at the Boston waterfront near the aquarium. Pigeons. Popcorn. Alexandra toddling. She can just about manage to hold a bag of popcorn in one hand while throwing kernels at the pigeons with the other. Delight.

Too soon, Alexandra reaches into the bag and discovers that there is no . . . more . . . popcorn. She is at first surprised, then clearly distressed. A moment later, she stoops down to the sidewalk, picks up a single kernel, and puts it carefully into the empty bag. She looks into the bag and says "Bye-bye," then looks away. She looks back into the bag at the single kernel of popcorn, says "Bye-bye," and is consoled. Unprepared for the end of her pigeon-and-popcorn adventure, Alexandra has devised a way to let go of the popcorn on her own terms. At sixteen months she is already learning to take care of herself. I am astonished and very glad.

A loving note penned a few months later by my dear friend Elissa, for the fete of my sixtieth birthday, concludes with this benediction: "May you always have the capacity to replace that last kernel in the bottom of your paper bag!"

Seventeen

Psychiatry and Beyond

*In the working genealogy of my profession, I am a direct de-*scendent (but not a fundamentalist disciple) of Sigmund Freud. My analyst had himself been analyzed by Dr. Grete Bibring, who had been analyzed by Freud. When I began my personal analysis I was thirty-one, had completed eight years of medical and psychiatric training, and felt ready for some professional independence. Analytic training at the Boston Psychoanalytic Institute would have meant signing on for eight additional years of "Mother, may I?" Semrad used to say, "The most important task of a human being is to make up his mind—what's for him and what's not for him." I knew that the inbred, stuffy, and controlling atmosphere of the Institute was not for me, and I chose to begin private practice, to arrange private supervision from senior psychiatrists I knew and respected, and to meet more informally for peer supervision with colleagues. I accepted an appointment to the faculty of Harvard's Massachusetts Mental Health Center, and I appreciated the vote of confidence in my work manifested by numbers of initial and ongoing referrals to my private practice by former supervisors.

My psychiatric office occupies more than half the ground floor of my three-story home. Private living space is upstairs, and I seldom spend time in the office when I am not working. Sometimes I refer to going down to the office to see patients as "going down to the salt mines," an epithet that connotes hard work, which it is, and drudgery, which—mostly—it is not; but, most aptly, it also connotes digging. Certainly, in terms of the patience, experience, care, and knowledge required, my work is more akin to archaeology than to what's associated with mining in Siberia.

A few times I've felt as though I've been in Siberia, though. I worked for a time with a woman who showed up depressed and unfulfilled by her life, lacking gusto for much of anything except for holding globally to a position of resentful compliance. During weekly sessions over a period of a couple of years, I tried everything I could think of—and I'm pretty resourceful—to create a nourishing place for her to grow. She did become considerably less depressed and more at peace with her life, but her self-centeredness was immovable. In our final session, with a bland expression on her face, she looked me in the eye and said: "I used to do what my mother wanted, to please my mother. Now I have to do what I want, to please *you*."

Such is this work, sometimes. Other times—truthfully and thankfully, most other times—what eventuates is considerably more full and satisfying.

What matters to my patients is, I believe, my commitment *to see it through* with them, whatever the issues may be. When first I meet a patient, the key matter is to find a point of common ground from which we can begin the work. One particular patient comes to present a challenge both figurative and literal. She is a woman in her late twenties who has been thrown out of therapy by her former psychiatrist, whom she stressed beyond that person's tolerance for bizarre behavior. At our first meeting, on entering the office, Emily sits down on the floor facing away from me and *behind* a chair, and does not speak. My office consists of two confluent rooms: a spacious consulting room, beyond which opens another room with bookcases, file cabinets, and a piano. At one point, Emily stands up and walks into the far room and to the right, out of my field of vision and in the vicinity of the file cabinets. The uncomfortable thought comes to me that she might be looking at patients' records. I call out to her: "Emily, are you looking in the files?"

Emily speaks for the first time, and in fury: "How dare you accuse me of looking in your files?"

I say, and not gently: "So, I was paranoid. You, of all people, can't understand and forgive that?"

We have found our common ground.

When we first meet, in the spring of 1979, Emily is physically healthy, psychotic, and does not want to live. When we say good-bye late in the summer of 1996, she is mentally clear, coping with cancer, and does not want to die. She has taught me most of what I know about psychosis—a lot, and over a major hunk of both our lives. She has learned well enough to manage her inside and outside world experience such that the sinister creatures she met in childhood (and can still see and hear if she chooses to pay attention to them) are no longer much of a factor in her life. Emily and I have both learned that for her psychosis is a set of symptoms that can be managed by the rest of the personality, if only that personality has what it needs to develop. Remarkably, she no longer uses any anti-psychotic medication at all.

Getting there was a long and at times harrowing journey. Early in the course of our work I realize that I will have to be clear with myself and honest with Emily as to the limits of what I can tolerate. She has already messed up several therapy relationships with other good doctors. Her symptoms are truly miserable. She has auditory hallucinations—something like several radio stations playing simultaneously in her head. Even in ninety-degree weather, she wears gloves and sweaters "to keep the molecules in." She lives with the conviction that she is an evil person and deserves to be punished. She has scars on her forearms from self-inflicted burns and slashes.

In the spirit of Semrad's observation:

No therapy is comfortable, because it involves dealing with pain. But there's one comfortable thought: that two people sharing pain can bear it easier than one . . .

I am prepared to be a partner to this anguished young woman, but I cannot inure myself to her self-mutilation. The bottom line: if she does not control her impulse to hurt herself, I will no longer work with her. It eventuates that Emily does not want me to quit, and however it comes to be so, she does not harm herself again. When, as happens intermittently for several years, she is desperate and cannot trust herself, she spends time on a psychiatric inpatient unit, where I continue as her doctor. We rely on the flexibly available and cooperative help of the inpatient and day hospital staff of a local hospital.

From the beginning, I prescribe antipsychotic medication. Emily systematically tries the lot of them, but regression to virtually unbearable psychosis regularly recurs. By midwinter 1983, we've been slogging through together for more than four years, and she is back in the hospital, miserably psychotic once again. Thankful that Emily is in good hands, and honestly glad for a break, I leave for vacation with Jenni, who is home from college. We'll have ten days in Maui, where I've rented an apartment with a lanai overlooking the Pacific.

Hawaii is magical: double rainbows nearly every day. Snorkeling not far from shore we see fish that rival the population of the Boston aquarium. From our terrace we watch whales breach and schools of porpoises arc across the water. Comparing our experience here to past visits to Pié de la Cuesta, in Mexico, the one thing we miss is flavorful food. Restaurant fare in Maui is, to our palates, pretty bland. Fortunately, we've got a kitchen, and I can make for market to provision a meal of spicy marinated chicken.

I want a whole chicken to roast, and I pass up the packages imported from the mainland in favor of what I assume is fresher local chicken. The native product does look a little weird. The chicken is ready to roast, but it has a very long neck still attached. This must be the Hawaiian way with chicken, I think, putting it into my shopping basket.

At the checkout, I am confused when I hear the clerk say *mahalo* to customer after customer. I've been intent on learning what few words present themselves in the Hawaiian language, and I've noticed the word *Mahalo* painted on public refuse containers. I've assumed this word to mean trash. Imagine my amusement to learn that *mahalo* is a word of blessing and thanks—"May you be in Divine breath."

Later that afternoon, while Jenni takes a Hawaiian siesta, I get the chicken into the oven and relax on the lanai with a book. I've brought several, have finished a novel, and have just started to read M. Scott Peck's *People of the Lie: The Hope for Healing Human Evil*. I had enjoyed this psychiatrist's first popular book, *The Road Less Traveled*, which described the challenges of life and of growth, and was written in well-articulated and familiar terms. I soon discover that this new book manifests something quite different. I find myself reading about patients whose symptoms Peck believes to be evidence of demonic possession, a condition to be cured only through the ritual of exorcism. I begin to feel creepy. I am thinking about Emily.

From time to time, I tear myself out of the book to check on dinner. Something is not quite right with this chicken. Not only does it have a long neck but, even after some time in the oven, it sits in the roasting pan looking kind of stiff. Compared to other chickens I have roasted, which seem to sort of relax as they cook, this chicken seems to be developing rigor mortis. Two hours later the chicken is still tough, and I am thoroughly spooked. My daughter wakes from her nap to find me in the act of tossing the chicken, which now I consider to be possessed, into the trash to be exorcised with the rest of the garbage. *Mahalo. Mahalo.* May we be in Divine breath.

I tell this anecdote lightly, and it is funny, but more soberly it is an example of the permeability of boundaries that made it possible for Emily and me to connect—and also with which I had to take care. Our relationship was one in which I lent Emily aspects of my ego—my capacity to cope (as when I interdicted her self-mutilation)—and in which I entered, carefully, into some aspects of her experience. Many of her fantasies were violent and disturbing, and at one point, when the dramatis personae included members of my family, I came finally to set a limit on what I was willing to hear. In this instance, in violation of a familiar paradigm, Emily was distinctly *not* free to tell her psychiatrist everything she was thinking. But it was in this way that she learned to take into account her impact on another person and her responsibility for respecting that person's tolerances. Eventually, and crucial to her growth, Emily learned to protect even herself from the disturbing elements that came into her own mind.

Two hours per week for seventeen years I did my best to help Emily to know herself, to accept and love herself, to manage herself, and occasionally even to enjoy herself, while, in the process, she came to know me and others, to tolerate being with me and others, and even occasionally to enjoy me and others. This was the work of psychotherapy. In Emily's life, knowing herself required tolerating noises in her head, weird discomfort in her body, and at times nearly unbearable chaos. Together we acknowledged what had to be borne, and tried to hold it as lightly as possible, to remain in the moment, and to let it go.

In my private practice of psychiatry, I have had the satisfying experience of "seeing it through" with hundreds of patients, a precious handful of whom were initially psychotic and eventually came no longer to qualify for this diagnosis. I have learned that while regression to overwhelming psychosis is caused by neurochemical imbalance, if a schizophrenic or manic-depressive patient has the roots of the capacity to relate to a skillful and committed therapist, and if the "fit" is a good one, with time and great effort, great gains are possible.

Common ground for connection is not much of a problem for most of the people who show up in my office. As true for me as for most of my patients (in Semrad's words):

> There are only a few choices in life: to kill yourself, go crazy, or learn to live with what you have in life.

The ways we go about trying not to have to accept what we have here and now and trying not to have to make peace with the past generate all kinds of what can be called neurotic suffering—pain that shows up as symptoms of anxiety, depression, obsessive thoughts, phobias, or physical malfunction.

When I am in my mid-thirties, and midway through my personal psychoanalysis, I learn something—the hard way—that proves useful both in my life and in my work with patients.

It happens like this. My daughter is at the cusp of adolescence, eleven years old and already taller than my five feet four. Shades of *Alice in Wonderland*, she has grown five inches this past year. The atmosphere of life these days feels something like it must down the rabbit hole. One day while we are shopping together and separately at the neighborhood supermarket, Jenni with one cart and I with another, I glance down as I pass an aisle, and see but do not immediately recognize my daughter, she has grown tall so quickly.

Until now I have been pretty relaxed about being a mother. Of late, seemingly from out of nowhere, I find myself at times frantic with worry about Jennifer. The occasions for anxiety have a common element: she is away for a day trip or an evening. What happens is that I'm okay for a while, but as the time for Jenni's return home approaches, I begin to be obsessed with the possibility that something dire may have happened to her. I suffer terribly with irrational thoughts verging on panic. Dependably, as soon as Jennifer is back, the whole miserable neurotic episode evaporates. That is, until the next time.

This will be Jenni's last summer at Green Acres, a nearby day camp she has attended for the past six years. Early in the summer she has an "overday"—a day when, instead of coming home in the afternoon, she and the other senior campers stay on for a campfire dinner. At about four o'clock that afternoon I begin to worry. I have to discipline myself not to drive to the camp to reassure myself that lions and tigers and bears have not this day invaded a Boston suburb. The moment my daughter arrives home in the evening, I'm fine, but I have been miserable with worry.

At the end of the summer, the last day of day camp for Jenni, ever, is marked by a couple of special events: her camp group's performance of their production of *Peter Pan* (in which Jenni plays Wendy and her best friend, Liz, plays Peter), followed by an overnight of camping. Parents are invited to the play. Of course I attend.

Sitting in the audience at the rustic outdoor amphitheatre, I watch the other groups of campers file in: the five-year-olds from Treetops, the six-year-olds from Brookside, the seven-year-olds from. . . . In my mind's eye, I see my little girl at five, at six, at seven. . . . The play begins, and there she is on stage, eleven years old, tall, and growing into womanhood. Too soon I am congratulating Jenni and the other kids and kissing my daughter good-bye—until tomorrow. There is, of course, that overnight.

Back in my car, I find myself overcome with sadness. No more Green Acres. No more little girl. Sobbing, my chest heaving, I have never before cried so deeply. I am left, finally, with a quieter sadness and an odd sense of peace. Still, as I drive home, I begin to gird against the irrational anxiety I expect to suffer this night.

But the panic never comes. In fact, it is never to come again. I have been taught a lesson about the genius of the unconscious. Its generation of neurotic pain functions as a distraction from the otherwise inevitable pain of living. At the time of my daughter's transition from childhood to adolescence, when I worried irrationally about some dire happening, I created a circumstance that was destined to have a happy ending. Again and again, as Jenni was restored safely to me, all my pain disappeared. This construct was an effective distraction from the reality that, day by day, my daughter was growing up and becoming increasingly independent. While of course I supported her growing independence, I could not avoid the sadness I felt at the ending of her childhood. Catalyzed by the event at Green Acres, when finally I succumbed to this sadness and wept, I no longer needed the distraction of the neurotic worry.

That's what Semrad meant by:

Life is really simple, but we don't let ourselves have it.

Having life means seeing what *is* and bearing the feelings that go with it. That is much of the work I do with my patients. The rest of it amounts to seeing what *was* and bearing the feelings that go with that. Another reminder of Semrad's observation regarding fruitless patterns:

The hope of the repetition compulsion:
that next time will be better!

I can't count the hours I've spent digging for the roots of patterns that my patients repeat, whose consequences they rue, and about which they complain. *How can this be happening to me? I'm furious*—this said when the outcome, given the pre-conditions, is predictable. It takes maturity and willingness to grieve in order to give up the futile effort of trying to change the past by repeating it with the determination to "fix it this time."

Patients often show up hoping *to get rid of* their anger, their sadness, their whatever. "Getting it out" is of use only in identifying what a person feels. There is no getting rid of anything. Integration is the word. The work, in Semrad's terms, is "to acknowledge, bear, and put into perspective" the facts and feelings of a person's life. Many of us resist recognizing that what's problematic about someone or something is often inseparably another aspect of what makes that person or circumstance valuable. Life's a package deal.

Over the decades since Freud, one psycho-something-or-other after the next has had its moment of limelight. Thomas Harris's *I'm OK—You're OK* was popular in the late 1960s and early 1970s. In my opinion, Elizabeth Kübler-Ross said it better: "I'm not okay, you're not okay, and that's okay." I have never been drawn to any modality that emphasizes one or a couple of aspects of anything. As a concept of life itself, the vitality of Zorba's "full catastrophe" can't be improved upon.

Just a few weeks before the pioneering feminist, teacher, and author Carolyn Heilbrun committed suicide, in the autumn of 2003, I was drawn in a bookstore to a collection of her essays entitled: *The Last Gift of Time: Life Beyond Sixty*. I was jolted to find, in the Preface, that she had "long ago settled upon the determination to end [her] life at seventy." I "met" her for the first time through this book, which I had picked up and put down several times, and finally read with a concentration and intensity unusual to my recent habit. Unusual for me, too, was a fantasy that came to me of meeting Heilbrun to consult about a patient with whom I was working who was conflicted about what might broadly be defined as "feminist issues."

On Friday, October 17, 2003, arriving early at Cape Cod to see a play by Sam Shepard that I had admired in reading but had never experienced on stage, I sat in my car at a spot overlooking the sea and finished the Heilbrun book. Just at that moment, my cell phone rang—my sweetheart phoning a hello and putting himself in line to hear the flow of ideas and responses stimulated by Heilbrun's essays. Our substantial connection of ten years is a blessing I had never dared dream of. He listened and then said, "You know she killed herself last week?" I had not known. Eerie. Had I in reading and fantasy for several days been unconsciously trying to keep this intellectually alive woman in the world? I felt something that vibrated to the frequency of that event of the October twenty-seven years earlier, when Semrad had died during a nap in his office. Ah . . . this universal power grid that cannot be explained by physics.

As chance would have it, recently I received an e-mail broadcast to Wellesley alumnae from the president of the college, Diana Chapman Walsh, to address the alumnae flap raised by the film *Mona Lisa Smile*, some of which was shot on location at the college. President Walsh described the film as "a Hollywood fantasy set in an imaginary 1953–1954 [Wellesley] academic year." On an impulse fueled in part by memories re-

vived in writing this memoir, I responded with the following
letter:

Dear President Walsh,

I attended Wellesley from 1957–1960.

Your letter evidences considerable comprehensive
understanding of the complexity of messy circumstances. If
only the Dean of the class of '61 had had such maturity and
wisdom. I consulted her about my conflict about leaving college
to marry. You may not believe it, but she told me not to make
the same mistake she had, or I'd end up an old maid.

At my 35th reunion, a fellow alumna and former dorm
mate told me that she had consulted the same dean about her
wish to go to medical school (a choice she subsequently
decided against and has since regretted). The dean advised
her <u>not</u> to go, as it would put undue financial hardship on her
family.

I <u>did</u> go to medical school—about which decision I had no
conflict, and so didn't offer it to the dean for comment.

. . . I trust that much has changed for the better in the
decades since. . . .

My best regards,
Susan Rako, M.D.

President Walsh replied:

Dear Dr. Rako:

In my ten years in the presidency, I have heard many
versions of the advice-from-the-dean story you tell here. Those
stories are all quite consistent with one another, and quite

inconsistent with what we, today, would consider helpful and appropriate counseling.

I believe and trust that our various counselors today . . . are creating a "holding environment" in which students can explore their options and dreams and find their own answers to life's complex questions, unencumbered by invasive advice and especially by advice that is contaminated with the personal projections and biases that seem so often to underlie the troubling stories we hear from earlier times.

I hope you've found many satisfactions in your medical career, a profession, it seems to me, that offers, more than most do, the possibility of finding that place where one's own deep gladness and the world's deep hunger meet, Frederick Buechner's definition of the idea of a "vocation."

Thanks for writing,
and best from Wellesley for the New Year,
Diana Walsh

So it happened that the backwash from a Hollywood movie opened a channel for the first warm feelings I experienced toward my alma mater in more than four decades.

I remember the convocation of my freshman class at Wellesley in September 1957. President Margaret Clapp's address to our class included an anecdote that went something like this:

As you go on with your education, you will find that you learn more and more about less and less until, when finally you know everything about nothing, you will have earned a Ph.D.

Amusing enough that I remember it, but hardly inspirational. A Zen master might make something more worthy than witty of this, but a Zen master Margaret Clapp was not. I am glad to have Diana Walsh's reference to Buechner to take its place as a quotable legacy from Wellesley.

I am now blessed with two vocations: the work of psychiatry and the work of educating women and their doctors about cutting-edge issues in women's reproductive health. Women's Health on Alert (WHOA), a newly founded charitable nonprofit organization for which I serve as president, has just received word of its first grant. Six months ago, WHOA was not even a dream—a hopeful reminder of the partnership of commitment and Providence. Now in my sixties, while integration and disintegration run neck and neck, I am glad to feel more whole and more freely myself even as my body increasingly expresses its age. I think about Semrad's adaptation of an old saw: "You can't win them all if you try; you can't win any of them if you don't," and I know that I am not ready to quit. Not by a long shot.

NOTES

Epigraph

Page 13   *"There is a crack"*   Leonard Cohen, "Anthem" from the album *The Future*, 1992, Sony.

Preface

Page 17   "Where id was, there ego shall be"   Sigmund Freud: "New Introductory Lectures in Psychoanalysis: Lecture XXXI: "The Dissection of the Psychical Personality," in *The Standard Edition of the Complete Psychological Works of Sigmund Freud*, ed. James Strachey (London: Hogarth Press, 1964), p. 80.

Page 18   "One becomes a therapist"   Susan Rako and Harvey Mazer, eds., *Semrad: The Heart of a Therapist* (New York: Jason Aronson Publishers, 1980; reissued Aronson and Scribner, 1983; reissued Lincoln, Neb.: iUniverse, 2003), p. 194. Citations are to the iUniverse edition.

Page 19   *The Hormone of Desire*   Susan Rako, *The Hormone of Desire: The Truth About Testosterone, Sexuality, and Menopause* (New York: Three Rivers Press, 1999).

Page 20   the research and writing of yet another   Susan Rako, M.D., *No More Periods? The Risks of Menstrual Suppression and Other Cutting-Edge Issues About Hormones and Women's Health* (New York: Crown, 2003).

Page 22   *Jung and the Story of Our Time*   Laurens van der Post, *Jung and the Story of Our Time* (New York: Pantheon, 1975).

Notes

Page 22   *Memories, Dreams, and Reflections*   C. J. Jung, recorded and edited by Aniela Jaffe, translated by Richard and Clara Winston (New York: Vintage Books, 1965).

One. Becoming

Page 37   "guilt is sometimes just guilt"   Fritz Perls, as quoted by Niela Miller in a Gestalt workshop, circa 1979.

Two. Mother, Music, and Me

Page 40   whose pupils had included Mischa Elman   Leopold Auer, *Violin Playing As I Teach It* (New York: Dover, 1980), back cover copy.

Page 42   my collection first of green-bound   Laura Lee Hope, The Bobbsey Twins Series (New York: Grosset & Dunlap, 1924).

Page 43   and later of blue-bound   Carolyn Keene, Nancy Drew Mystery Stories (New York: Grosset & Dunlap, 1936).

Page 43   the title of one of her favorites   Marguerite Steen, *The Sun Is My Undoing* (New York: Viking Press, 1942).

Page 47   *The Red Shoes*   Directed by Michael Powell and Emeric Pressburger, 1948.

Page 53   Leonard Bernstein's piano teacher   Gerald Martin Bordman, *American Musical Theatre: A Chronicle,* 3rd ed. (New York: Oxford University Press, 2001), p. 599.

Page 57   for the launch of my new book   Rako, *No More Periods?*

Four. About God

Page 64   "Follow that will and that way"   Carl Jung, letter to Miguel Serrano, September 14, 1960, in *Letters, Vol. 2: 1951–1961,*

ed. Gerhard Adler (Princeton: Princeton University Press, 1975), p. 592.

Page 72   *"When our children feel"*   Aron Hirt-Manheimer, ed., *The Jewish Condition: Essays on Contemporary Judaism Honoring Rabbi Alexander M. Schindler* (New York: UAHC Press, 1995), p. 362.

Page 72   *"Words like despair"*   Ibid., p. 401.

Page 79   *A Matter of Heart*   *A Matter of Heart: The Extraordinary Journey of C. G. Jung into the Soul of Man,* documentary film on VHS, directed by Mark Whitney (Los Angeles: C. G. Jung Institute of Los Angeles, 1983).

Page 82   interpretation of the *I Ching*   Carol B. Anthony, *A Guide to the I Ching* (Stow, Mass.: Anthony Publishing Company, 1988).

Five. Alone, Together, Alone

Page 89   *"The more mature a relationship"*   Rako, *Semrad,* p. 48.
Page 89   *"You can only be close"*   Ibid., p. 49.

Six. Scientific Foundations

Page 92   in my book of fables and morality tales   Watty Piper, ed., "The Stone in the Road" in *Folk Tales Children Love* (New York: Platt and Munk, 1932).

Seven. Medical School—Married and Pregnant

Page 108   a novel that had until recently been banned   D. H. Lawrence, *Lady Chatterley's Lover* (New York: Grove Press, 1957).

Notes

Page 109 the story of my pregnancy   Vivian Cadden, "A Husband's Diary of His Wife's Pregnancy," *Redbook*, June 1964.

Page 111 *"The moment one definitely commits"*   William H. Murray, *The Scottish Himalayan Expedition* (London: J. M. Dent & Sons, 1951), pp. 6–7.

Ten. Transitions

Page 127 *"When you use a hospital"*   Rako, *Semrad*, p. 182.

Page 127 "May I have your permission"   Ibid., p. 134.

Page 128 experienced psychiatrists and trainees alike   Ibid., pp. 11–12.

Eleven. Psychiatric Residency

Page 136 "just a hayseed from Nebraska"   Rako, *Semrad*, p. 12.

Page 136 *"The first year, the experience"*   Ibid., p. 186

Page 136 *"As a psychiatrist"*   Ibid., p. 105.

Page 136 *"Laymen often think"*   Ibid., p. 106.

Page 136 *"A man's either scared"*   Ibid., p. 115.

Page 137 *"Symptoms are solutions"*   Ibid., p. 163.

Page 137 *"Normality is essentially"*   Ibid., p. 87.

Page 137 *"Falling in love is"*   Ibid., p. 33.

Page 139 *to investigate, investigate*   Ibid., p. 110.

Page 144 *"I've never seen a group"*   Ibid., p. 180.

Page 144 *"We're in an era"*   Ibid., p. 180.

Page 144 the writings of the British psychiatrist   Ronald D. Laing, *The Divided Self* (New York: Pantheon, 1960), and *The Politics of Experience* (New York: Pantheon, 1967).

Page 144 and an American psychiatrist   Thomas Szasz, *The Myth of Mental Illness* (New York: Harper & Row, 1961).

Page 145 *symptoms are solutions*   Rako, *Semrad*, p. 163.

Notes

Page 145   drawn to the writings of   Donald W. Winnicott, *Playing and Reality* (New York, Basic Books, 1971).

Page 147   *"Sorrow is the vitamin"*   Rako, *Semrad*, p. 45.

Page 148   "How did you make him"   Ibid., p. 133.

Twelve. Second Marriage

Page 151   "Everyone has to buy peace"   Rako, *Semrad*, p. 23.

Page 152   "The hope of the repetition compulsion"   Ibid., p. 155.

Fourteen. Finding My Father

Page 168   "the full catastrophe"   *Zorba the Greek*, 1964 screenplay by Michael Cacoyannis adapted from the novel by Nikos Kazantzakis (New York: Simon & Schuster, 1901).

Page 169   *"The only way a father"*   Rako, *Semrad*, pp. 53–54.

Page 169   *"Every time you put a mile"*   Ibid., p. 53.

Sixteen. True Reflection

Page 180   *The Child, the Family, and the Outside World*   Donald W. Winnicott, *The Child, the Family, and the Outside World* (Harmondsworth: Penguin, 1964).

Page 181   "the squiggle game"   Donald W. Winnicott, *Therapeutic Consultations in Child Psychiatry* (New York: Basic Books, 1971).

Seventeen. Psychiatry and Beyond

Page 184   "The most important task"   Rako, *Semrad*, p. 76.

Page 187   *"No therapy is comfortable"*   Ibid., p. 106.

Notes

Page 189   have just started to read   M. Scott Peck, *People of the Lie* (New York: Simon & Schuster, 1983).

Page 189   this psychiatrist's first popular book   M. Scott Peck, *The Road Less Traveled* (New York: Simon & Schuster, 1978).

Page 191   *"There are only a few choices"*   Rako, *Semrad,* p. 80.

Page 194   *"Life is really simple"*   Ibid., p. 97.

Page 194   *"The hope of the repetition compulsion"*   Ibid., p. 155.

Page 195   "acknowledge, bear, and"   Ibid., p. 104.

Page 195   I was drawn in a bookstore   Carolyn Heilbrun, *The Last Gift of Time* (New York: Ballantine Books, 1998).

Page 198   the place where one's own deep gladness   Frederick Buechner, *Wishful Thinking* (San Francisco: Harper, 1993), p. 119.

Page 199   "You can't win them all"   Rako, *Semrad,* p. 78.

PERMISSIONS

ABOUT THE AUTHOR

Following medical education at Albert Einstein College of Medicine and specialty training in psychiatry at Harvard's Massachusetts Mental Health Center, Dr. Rako established an active private psychiatric practice in Newton, Massachusetts, more than thirty years ago, which she continues to serve and to enjoy. Her groundbreaking book, *The Hormone of Desire: The Truth About Testosterone, Sexuality, and Menopause*, has brought her to international prominence as an authority in the field of women's reproductive health. In 2003 she founded the educational nonprofit *Women's Health on Alert, Inc. (WHOA)*.

On a parallel track with her medical work, Dr. Rako earned an M.S. in film production in 1988 from Boston University College of Communication. In May 2005, as executive producer, she brought the Boston premier of the play *Hysterics* to the Lyric Stage.

Dr. Rako can be reached through her website, www.susanrako.com.